Herbal Cream Making

A guide to botanical balms, creams and lotions

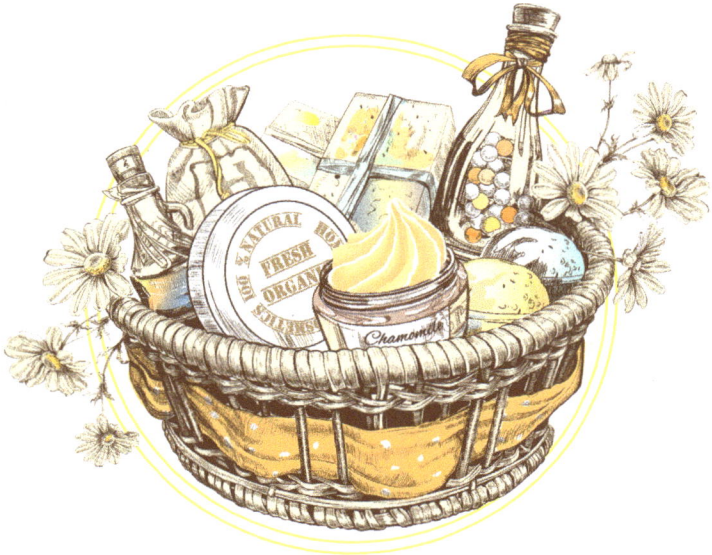

Dawn Ireland

Herbal Cream Making

The information contained in this book is presented for interest only. Neither Herbary Books nor the author accept any liability relating to the use of this information. Please consult your medical herbalist or physician if you are unsure about following any of the advice in this book.

ISBN 978-1-9163396-9-9

HERBARYBOOKS

Published by Herbary Books
Caernarfon, Wales
www.herbarybooks.com
contact@herbarybooks.com

Contents

Introduction	1
The art and science of cream making	8
What is a cream?	10
Patch testing and allergies	13
Equipment	15
Basic Equipment	16
The boundary: All about the skin	18
Structure and function of the skin	20
PH matters	20
Two influences on skin health	22
Layers of the skin	23
Dermal absorption	24
Preservation	25
Water solubles	26
Fat solubles	27
Manufactured preservatives	28
Allergens	29
What makes a cream?	30
Building layers of botanicals for the most effective product	32
Hydrosols	33
Teas	35
Glycerites	36
Macerated oils	36
Tinctures	37
Fresh plant juice	38
Essential oils	38
CO^2 extracts	39
Macerated solid fats	40
Fixed or Carrier oils	40

Fats and butters 42
    Plant waxes 44
    Emulsifiers 45

Skin care herbs 48

Yarrow *(Achillea millefolium)* 50
Horse chestnut/conker *(Aesculus hippocastanum)* 51
Aloe Vera *(Aloe vera)* 52
Marshmallow *(Althaea officinalis)* 53
Bearberry *(Arctostaphylos uva-ursi)* 54
Oats *(Avena sativa)* 55
Daisy *(Bellis perennis)* 56
Barberry/Oregon Grape *(Berberis vulgaris and Berberis aquifolium)* 57
Pot marigold *(Calendula officinalis)* 58
Chilli pepper *(Capsicum spp.)* 60
German & Roman chamomile *(Chamomilla recutita & Anthemis nobilis)* 62
Greater celandine *(Chelidonium majus)* 63
Myrrh sap resin *(Commiphora myrrha)* 64
Turmeric *(Curcuma longa)* 65
Meadowsweet *(Filipendula ulmaria)* 66
Bladderwrack seaweed *(Fucus vesiculosis)* 67
Wintergreen *(Gaultheria procumbens)* 68
Liquorice *(Glycyrrhiza glabra)* 69
Witch hazel *(Hammamelis virginiana)* 70
St. John's Wort *(Hypericum perforatum)* 70
Lemon balm *(Melissa officinalis)* 71
Peppermint *(Mentha piperita)* 72
Rosemary *(Rosmarinus officinalis (Salvia rosmarinus))* 73
Plantain *(Plantago spp.)* 74
Milk thistle *(Silybum marianum/Carduus marianus)* 75
Chickweed *(Stellaria media)* 76
Comfrey *(Symphytum officinalis)* 77
Thyme *(Thymus vulgaris)* 78

Recipes for creams, lotions, balms and salves 80

Gentle salve ointment 84

Whipped balm butter   85
Thick cream   86
Light cream   88
Lotion   90
Mousse-type lotion   92
Thin emulsion-type lotion   93
Aloe gel   94

Dawn's favourite herb and cream combinations   96
for common conditions

Antiseptic cream   98
Bruise cream   98
Chest balm salve   99
Dermatitis anti-inflammatory cream   100
Eczema cream or lotion   100
Fungicidal cream   101
Gentle healing balm   102
Keratosis cream   103
Melasma cream   104
Pain relief cream   104
Psoriasis cream   105
Salve for split fingers & gardener's   106
hand protection
Sunburn lotion   107
Varicose vein lotion   108
Wart remover cream   108

Troubleshooting   110

Further reading   114
Latin and common names of plants   116
Bibliography   117
Suppliers of ingredients   118
References   119

About the author   125

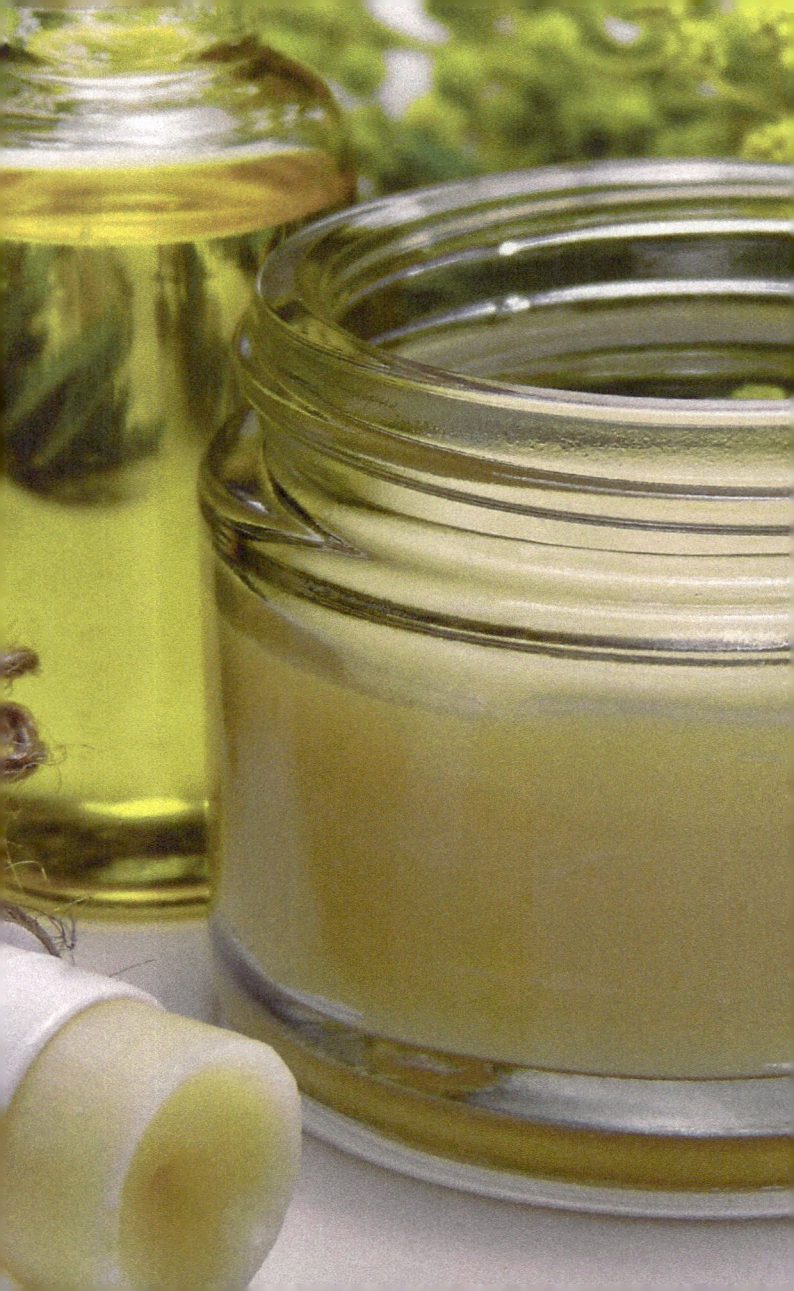

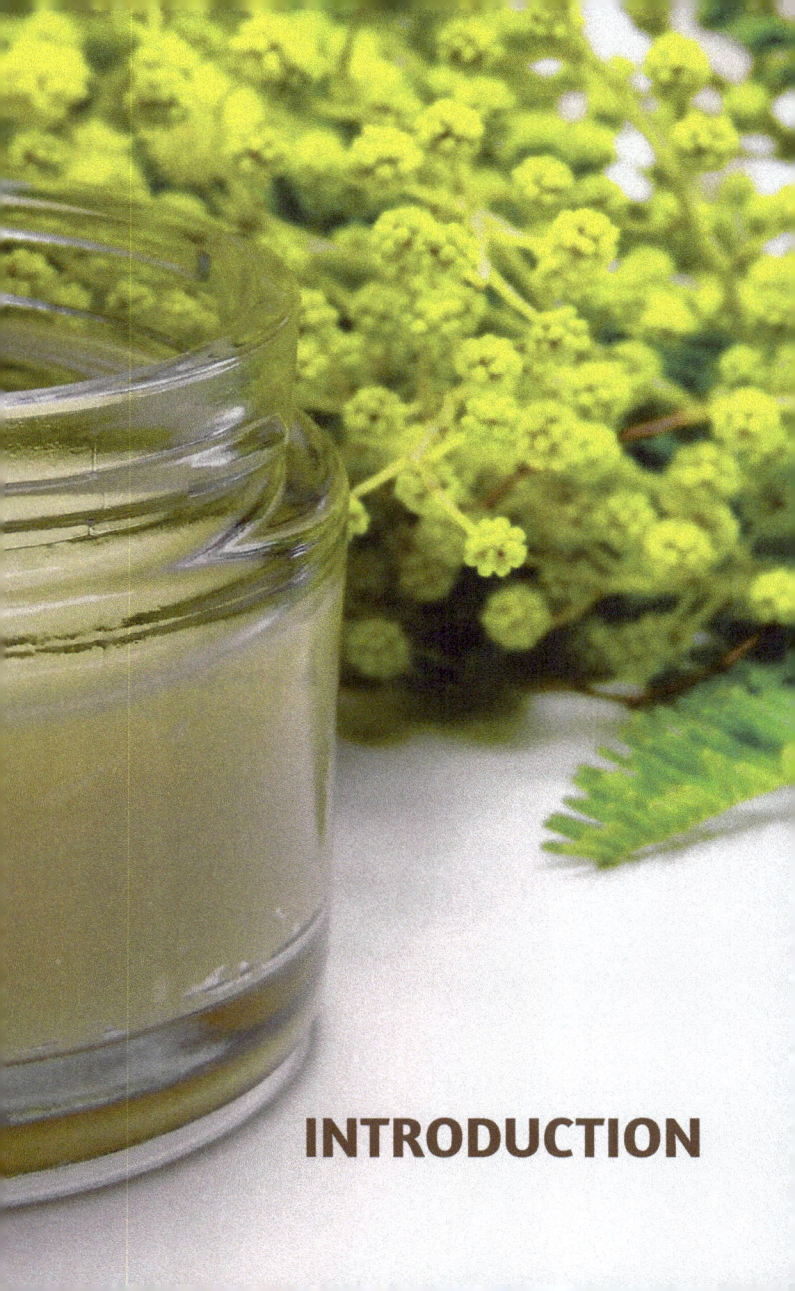

INTRODUCTION

The first time you successfully make a cream or lotion feels like magic, proper potion making alchemy. The blending and mixing of waters and oils to make a beautiful, smooth, skin friendly, healing, herbal product is a skill you can adapt to your own preferences for anything you need, and more enjoyable than buying ready-made.

I grew up with my grandparents who instilled in me a love of books and of plants, and who suffered my childhood potion making activities with benign acceptance, much as my husband does today, treating each dish or jar stored in the fridge with understandable suspicion and the question asked 'is this food or not?'

For me the whole point of making my own creams originally was to control the ingredients and make creams with botanical extracts that weren't available in the shops. My aim was to avoid harsh chemical and artificial additives and to make full use of the wonderful botanicals available. I had disasters and mistakes along the way: that is how you learn. My first really successful cream was lavender and comfrey, thick but non greasy, smelled amazing, went on smoothly with a wonderful feeling on the skin. I shared it around my friends and neighbours. Then three days later it grew a thick fuzzy coat of fur, it had gone mouldy. Then I started learning about preservation.

I first began making creams properly around 2001: initially for my own use, then for friends and family. I had no relevant training or qualifications at that point. I had a couple of books and learned by trial and error, and lots of research. In my past career, I spent a few bored years working in office environments and knew it wasn't for me. My journey into herbalism began when I took a couple of courses on using herbs medicinally, and growing them. In those days it was by correspondence courses. I volunteered at a local charity trust in a heritage walled garden and learned a huge amount about gardening and was given several herb borders to design myself. Then I took a diploma in Iridology, and was introduced to a holistic college in Torquay (Kevala Centre, sadly no longer there) and was asked to run some workshops on making basic products. I expanded these workshops to other local groups, and took a diploma in teaching adult education classes. I set up making and selling a basic skin care range in 2003 (Green Wyse) making organic and therapeutic cosmetics. From here it was a natural progression to undertake a degree (BSc) in Herbal Medicine and aim to move my career

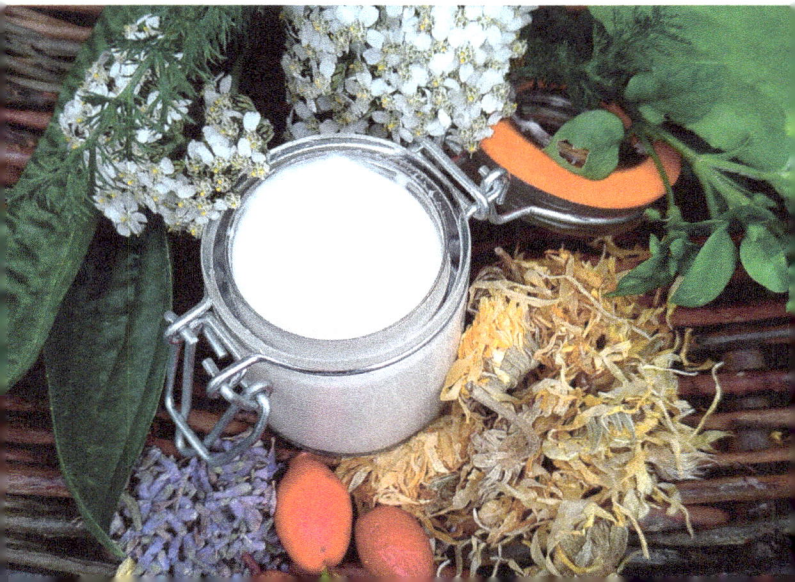

fully into holistic health. Since graduating in 2011 and setting up my herbal medicine practice in Torquay, (torbay-herbalist) I have also studied a short course in Plant Based Nutrition with Winchester University, and achieved a diploma with Formula Botanica in Advanced Cosmetic Science. For a couple of years I taught herbal remedies for home use at my local college of further education. I have taught herbal pharmacy practical skills on the Betonica School of Herbal Medicine course.

I grow many herbs myself, and make a lot of my own herbal medicines. It's surprising how much you can grow in a tiny town garden. By no means is my learning journey into herbal and natural product making complete, and it never will be. I don't know everything, and the information given here is simply what I have tried and found to be effective, and I apologise in advance if any errors are found. I don't consider myself a natural academic, but I have researched and included references when possible, although it should be remembered that sometimes we don't know why a herb works as it does, it's simply knowledge from generations upon generations of effective use. Traditional knowledge

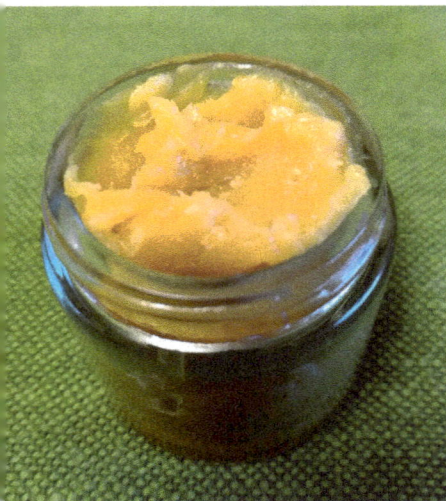

Daisy bruise balm

should not be dismissed; herbs are more than a range of chemical constituents. Modern science has now begun to show why certain herbs work for certain conditions, analysing constituents and working with clinical trials. I have included some human relevant studies, in vitro cell analysis and human clinical trials.

This guide is designed for both beginners and for experienced formulators and herbalists, everyone will hopefully learn something. The recipes or formulas can be made into cosmetic or medicinal products by switching around ingredients. It is ideal for those wishing to avoid artificial and synthetic ingredients, for those with allergies who need control over content, for those wishing to make products better than those you can buy, and for those keen on being as plastic free, and zero waste as possible. The guide starts with explanations of ingredients, techniques and troubleshooting, with some tried and tested techniques and formulas or recipes you can easily make with the reassurance they will work. Some information on herbs, plants and botanical extracts is included with benefits to the skin and a few basic skin conditions. A list of resources, how to process your own plant material or where to buy is also included. Once you have the techniques you can create your own bespoke products. This guide does not cover the legalities about selling products to the public.

The skin is often described as a mirror of internal health, and certainly many systemic conditions manifest in skin symptoms.

Many herbs work quickly, however, in my experience, most work gradually, building up slowly over a period of time. We have become impatient in our world of instant results, and I believe it is important to emphasise working with the body using natural methods shouldn't be expected to produce results straight away. For instance a commercial anti-fungal cream which might show results in as little as two days, but potentially cause side effects both to the user and the environment[1], when replaced by a herbal cream it may take many days to start taking effect. Not only this but perhaps needs using twice or three times daily alongside excellent hygiene, shoe sterilisation (UV light is best, natural or electric shoe inserts) and then to be continued for quite a few weeks afterwards to maintain the benefits, alongside internal treatment for the reason it was able to get a hold, such as too much sugar in the diet for instance. Having said that, herbal pain relief creams can often work quicker and be more effective than any over the counter preparations.

Image right. Turmeric and Greater Celandine cream

1 Drugs.com. 'Canesten Side Effects: Common, Severe, Long Term'. https://www.drugs.com/sfx/canesten-side-effects.html.

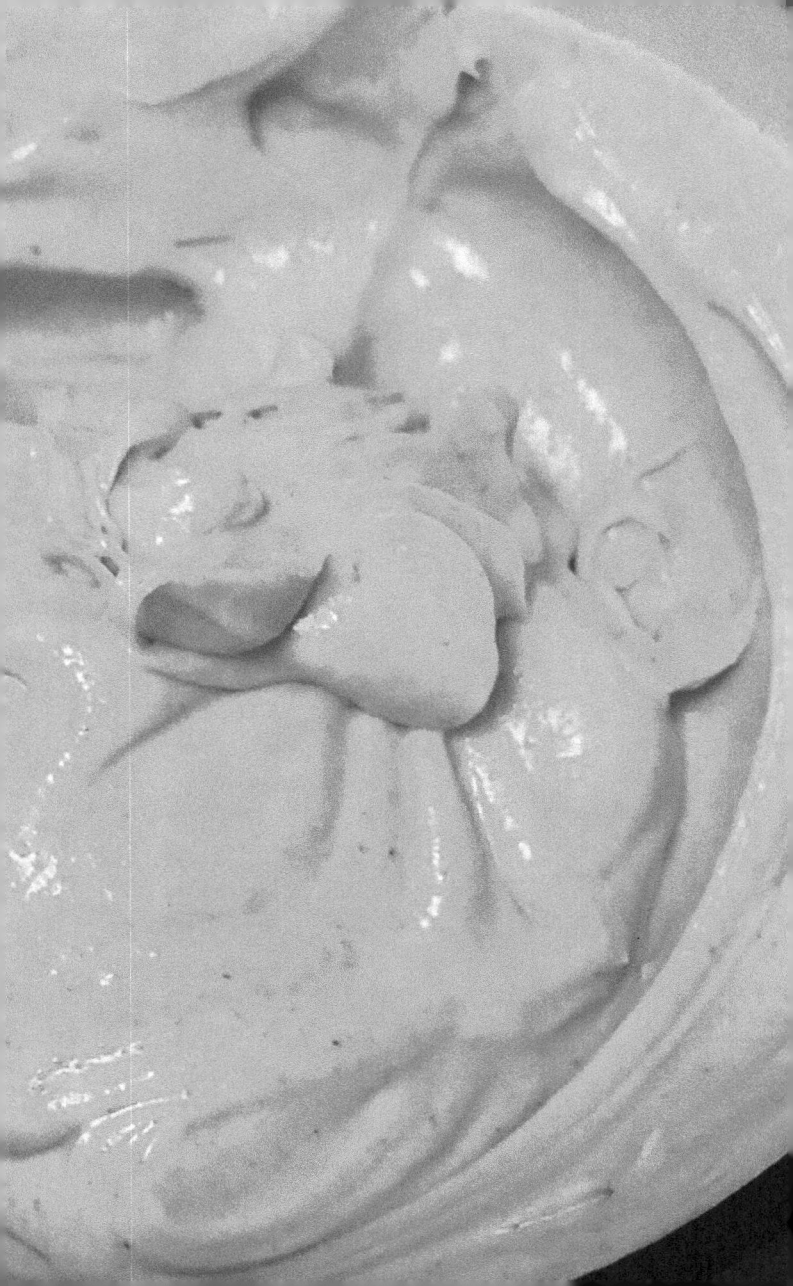

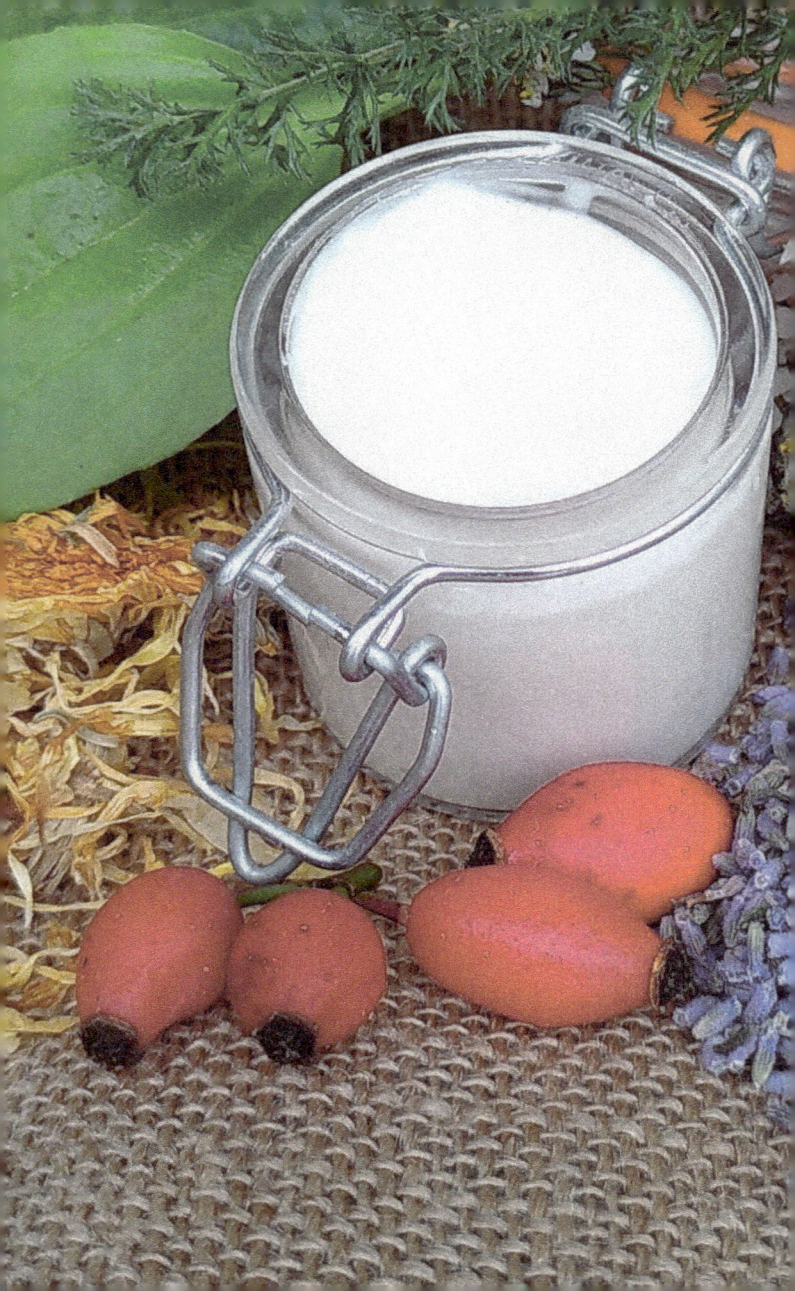

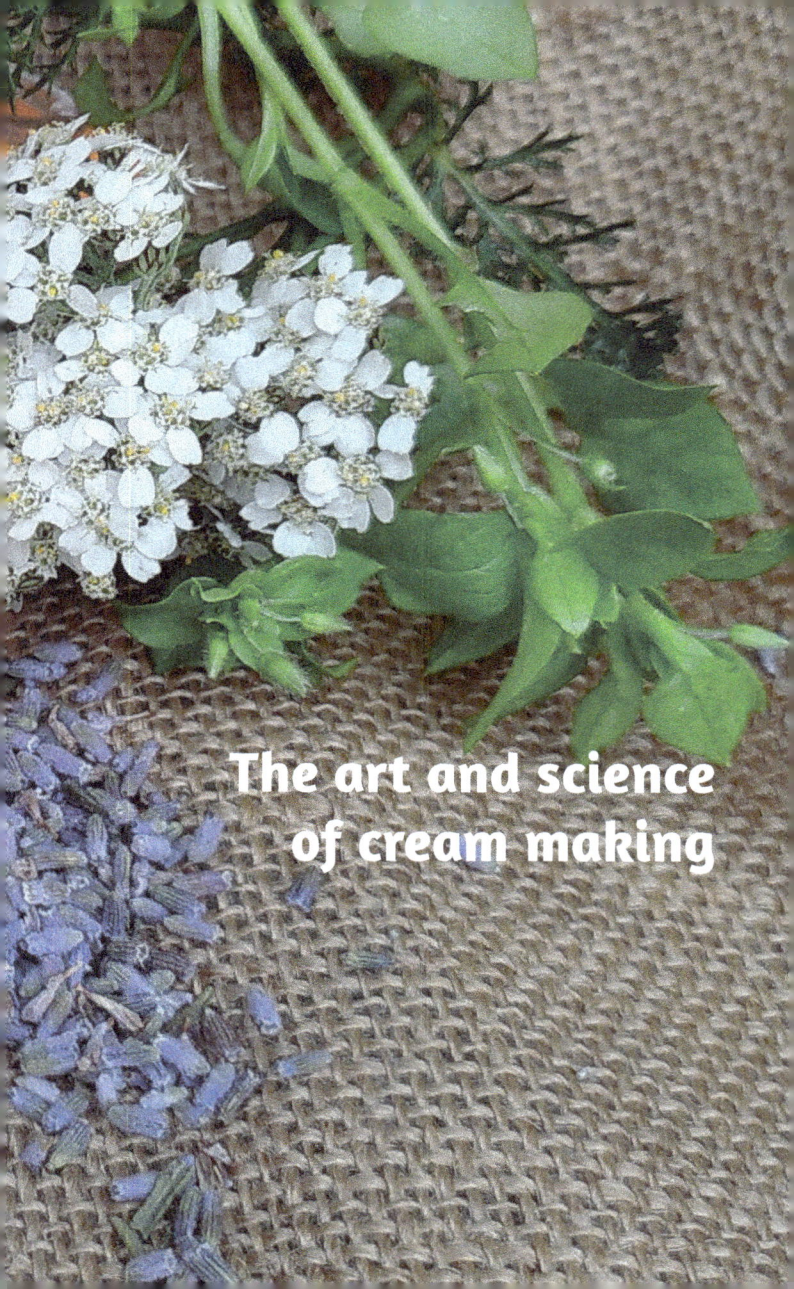

The art and science
of cream making

What is a cream?

Labels and names can be misleading. Strictly speaking a cream must be a combination of water soluble and oil soluble ingredients, blended together and held together, or emulsified.

Ointments, balms, and salves should consist only of oils, fats and waxes and contain no watery ingredients at all. Gels are usually only water-soluble ingredients, but can sometimes contain a small proportion of oil solubles, or essential oils for instance. However, you will find many products called ointments or butters which are actually thick creams. The only way to be sure is to read the label. The only reason this may matter, is your treatment aim.

Fat based preparations include ointments, salves, balms and butters and contain fat soluble, or lipophilic ingredients. (Lipo meaning fat, philic meaning 'to like'). They generally sit on the surface of the skin or upper layers of the skin and form a barrier. They are useful at protecting the skin from the outside world as they seal in moisture, prevent drying and protect from dirt and damp: For instance nappy ointments, gardeners hand balms and lip salves. They are also useful from a herbalist's point of view for encouraging someone to massage an area which may be part of the therapy, such as arthritic knees or wrists which may benefit from improving circulation which means nutrients delivered and metabolic wastes cleared more efficiently through the bloodstream. The individual components will slowly release into the top layers of the skin, and for pain relieving balms this can be helpful for slow release analgesia with essential oils such as wintergreen where components such as the salicylate glycosides maintain pain relief over a period of a few hours[2]. Essential oils are usually neither an oil or a water but something of both. Some of the constituents of the essential oil will therefore gain access to the deeper tissues over a period of time as a salve melts into the top layers of skin. Oils are usually liquid at room temperature, solid fats such as coconut oil, cocoa butter and shea butter have various melting temperatures and are usually solid at room temperature in the northern hemisphere, waxes remain solid at higher temperatures and are often sold in pellet form.

Creams and lotions are very user friendly, being a blend of both waters and oils; they absorb easily and are lighter and easier to apply than salves. They relay their ingredients into the deepest skin layers quickly: water

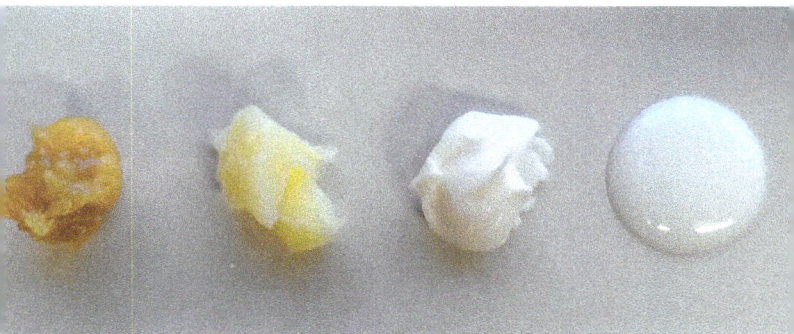

Image above. Left to right: salve, whipped butter, thick cream, lotion

2 Martin, et. al. 'Dermal Absorption of Camphor, Menthol, and Methyl Salicylate in Humans'. *J. Clin. Pharmacol* 44, no. 10: 1151–57.

contents initially, then oily contents. They leave a non-greasy protective film on the skin.

Gels are popular for quick applications where only the top layer of the skin needs to be treated. They are helpful in early stages of sunburn, such as aloe and lavender, or peppermint cooling gel for heat rash.

Emulsifiers are substances that have a molecular structure with lipophilic (fat liking) and hydrophilic (water liking) opposite ends. So one end attaches to the water solubles, and one end attaches to the fat solubles and binds them together. Think of making mayonnaise in the kitchen, vinegar is the hydrophilic ingredient, then oil which is lipophilic, then the egg yolk which is a natural emulsifier as it contains lecithin. In cream making for cosmetics and medicinal products, there are many emulsifiers. Some are derived from petrochemicals and can be irritating and drying on the skin. Some are natural such as lecithin extracted from sunflower seeds or soya beans, and some are in between, extracts made in a lab but from natural bases so are skin friendly in their own right. The end result of the product will be very different according to which is used. An emulsifier can be used in balms, salves and ointments to create a smooth product even though there are no hydrophilic

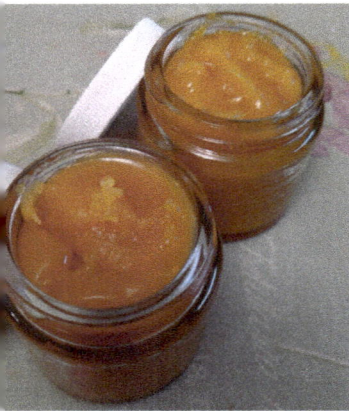

Image above. Calendula salve

ingredients. It is possible to make balms without an emulsifier, by vigorous whipping of ingredients together as it cools and thickens with the right ratio of oils, fats and waxes. However, without an emulsifier there is always the risk that in warm temperatures some fatty acids will melt, and others remain solid, causing your balm to become gritty and lumpy. The troubleshooting section will explain how to address this.

The hydrophilic portion of a cream can be plain water, herb tea, hydrosol (sometimes called hydrolats) such as rosewater or witch hazel – a distilled product. Be aware of the difference between a pure hydrosol and a floral water which may be plain water, essential oil and a chemical dispersant. The label will confirm the content.

The basic method of making a cream is to warm or melt some lipophilic and hydrophilic ingredients to a formula or recipe, in separate containers, achieving the same temperatures, adding an emulsifier and then blending together. Just like cooking. If you are learning from scratch, start simple and build up. Always remember, making mistakes is how you learn, there is no such thing as a failure, it's a learning step.

Patch testing and allergies

A note on patch testing and allergies. It is sensible to take some precautions. Just because herbs and plant based ingredients are natural, it does not mean to say they are suitable for everyone and natural substances can cause irritation and allergic reactions. It is recommended you carry out a patch test with every product you create. Take a small amount of the product and rub into the skin on the inside of your wrist or elbow. Leave for 24 hours and check for any reaction. If the skin becomes red, itchy, swollen or sore, caution is needed. You could then narrow things down by trying each ingredient of that product, one at a time, in another patch test to see which one caused the problem, with the exception of essential oils and CO_2 extracts which usually shouldn't be used neat on the skin. If you get an immediate strong reaction, wash off immediately with soap and water and seek help if needed. Essential oils have maximum safe dermal limits, more on this in the resources section.

Keep a diary or notebook. I learned to my cost that you will not remember the exact measurements of a recipe. When you begin to experiment, adding a little of this or that, you need to be sure you can repeat it when the result is the best cream you've ever made.

Try to use organic ingredients whenever possible. It seems a shame to go to the trouble of creating your own products and use non organic materials. Pesticide residues from food we eat and air we breathe have been proven to end up in body tissues, breast milk and are often endocrine disruptors[3]. In other words, they could have a negative influence on all the hormones in your body and your immune system. This goes for the products we use on our skin, a proportion of which are absorbed, and for our household cleaners and fragrancers. Go natural

3 Mnif et al, 2011, 'Percutaneous Absorption Enhancers: Mechanisms and Potential'. *Brazil Arch. Biol & Technol*. 50, no. 6 949–61

whenever possible, it is better for us and for wildlife and the planet as a whole. What we wash off our skin goes down the drain into the water table. Sometimes organic may be unavailable, but the more we request it, the more likely producers and growers are to identify and meet the demand.

Equipment

Most of the equipment you will need can be borrowed from your kitchen, or as many herbalists like to say 'a herbalists kitchen is full of equipment not used for its original purpose'. Glass, pyrex, ceramic, steel and enamel are easily cleaned leaving no residual scent. Plastics are best kept separate for kitchen and cream making uses as they can retain scents from both food and essential oils. If you are selling products you are advised to keep a separate set of equipment from kitchen utensils. Avoid using aluminium, cast iron uncoated or non-stick coated pans as they may all leach compounds into your product. A bain-marie or double boiler is a pan which sits on top of another pan which is half filled with water. An alternative is a heat proof bowl placed in a pan of water. This avoids overheating or burning when melting fats and heating oils. When you remove the pan or bowl, carefully wipe the bottom to avoid water drips getting into your product. You can also place a cloth between the bowl and pan if it sits too low, to stop direct contact. It is also quite possible to make creams just using two small pans directly on the hotplate, as long as you are very careful not to allow overheating. The oils particularly heat up very quickly, so vigilance is needed.

Basic equipment

- Bain-marie, double boiler pan or heat proof bowl/jug with small pan
- Measuring beakers or jugs
- Tablespoons
- Teaspoons
- Accurate weighing scales
- Sieve or strainer (metal is best)
- Containers for finished products – glass are my favourite as they can be sterilised and reused
- Thermometer, either a glass one or a contact free infrared cooking type (the latter is one of my favourite items as it avoids the dripping of oils and waters as you measure and move between pans)
- Spatulas – silicone are my favourite
- Whisks, hand or electric – mini balloon hand whisks are great for small batches, or mini coffee foam blenders, stick blenders for larger batches
- PH testing strips or meter

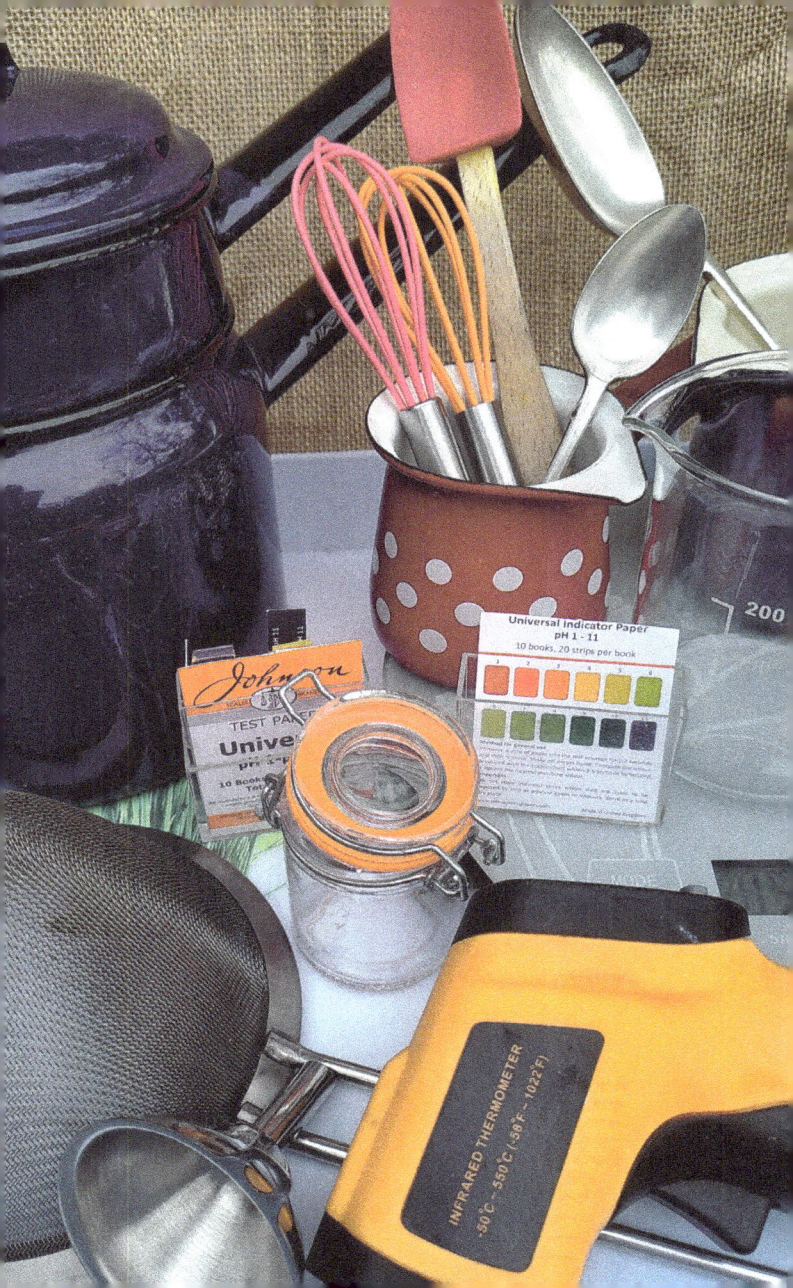

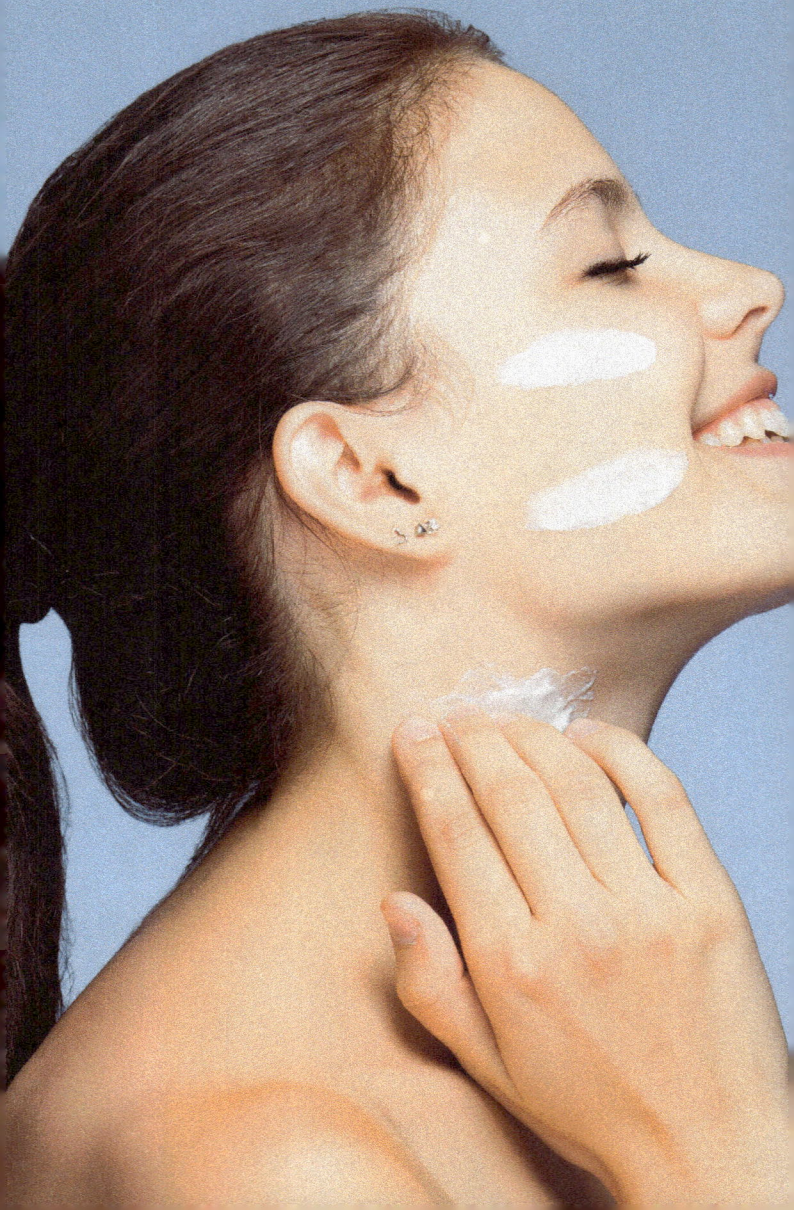

The boundary:
All about the skin

- Protection of inner tissues. The skin has resident immune cells, for defence and attack of external pathogens. In the event of an insult, the skin-resident immune cells are also involved in tissue reconstruction.
- Temperature regulation. Nerve endings send messages and keep a constant vigil of external conditions and react accordingly with methods such as raising hairs to trap warmth, flattening them to reduce heat, contracting and expanding capillaries, and sweating.
- Sensation messaging is sent via pressure receptors to protect from pain and potentially damaging insults to the skin and tissues and to help with proprioception, the sense of where your body is placed such as feet on the ground.
- As an organ of elimination the skin is used for excretion of small amounts of metabolic wastes such as urea, cortisol, salt, potassium and uric acid.
- Metabolism of vitamin D on exposure to UVB light
- Host to a population of beneficial bacteria which fight the pathogenic ones we are challenged with.

PH matters

The maintenance of good health is dependent on keeping pH levels balanced. Neutral on the scale being 7, lower than that is towards acidity, higher is towards alkalinity. Different tissues and fluids in the body need slightly different levels, such as the stomach needing high acidity to digest food and kill food pathogens. The skin has optimum pH levels slightly on the acidic side around 5.5 over most of the body[4]. This maintains an efficient barrier, promotes populations of friendly bacteria and enzymes, maintains flexibility, reduces dryness, and is hostile to pathogenic bacteria and fungal growth.

Natural soap, cleansers and detergents are usually alkaline to enable them to work efficiently. Some synthetic detergent cosmetics and soap like bars 'syndets' have a lower pH, however, the use of synthetic detergents has been shown to be detrimental to the skin. Use of these often means the skin is left dry, itchy and has that tight feeling. Using mildly acidic products following washing re-establishes the 'acid mantle' condition of the skin. If you have ever tried a vinegar rinse following shampooing you will know how soft and shiny this makes your hair, just a tablespoon in a

4 Ali, S, and G Yosipovitch. 'Skin PH: From Basic SciencE to Basic Skin Care'. *Acta Dermato Venereologica* 93, no. 3: 261–67

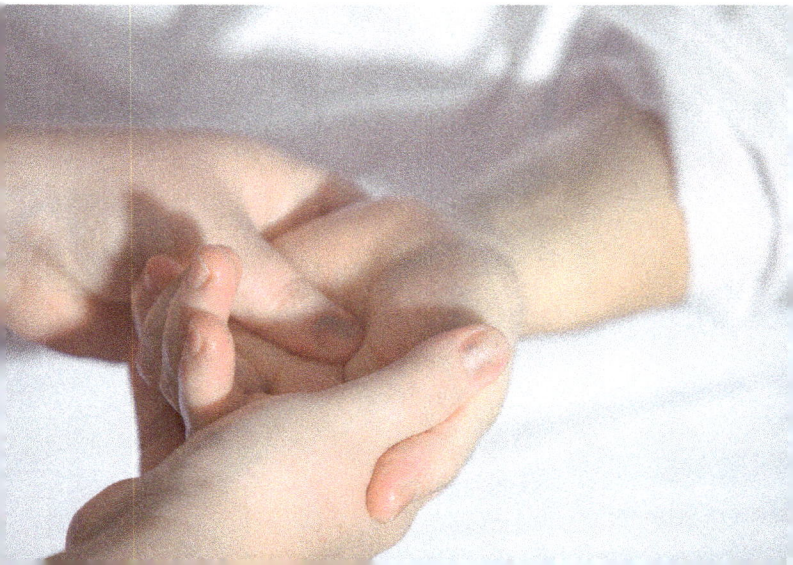

pint of rinsing water is enough to smooth down the cuticles on the hair shaft, creating silky easy to comb hair. The skin benefits from use of a cream or lotion with a pH between 4 and 6 whether this is cosmetic or medicinal. Maintenance of the integrity of your skin will stand you in good stead for healing of wounds, and combats tissue fragility. When you make your own products you can control the pH. Testing a formula when you experiment to get this right is worth doing, once you have it, you know when you repeat the same recipe, the pH will be the same. You can also adjust the pH during the process by adding a tiny bit of citric acid, lemon juice or vinegar to lower pH, or a little bicarbonate of soda to increase (a pinch or a few drops only).

Two influences on skin health are

- Exogenous (from the outside world) – pollution, injury, infection, excessive UV exposure, harsh cleansing products
- Endogenous (from inside) – malnutrition, ageing, illness, dehydration, some medications

As we age microcirculation becomes less efficient, collagen and elastin (underlying structures plumping up skin tissues) reduce and become less ordered. pH levels slowly rise, sebum production decreases, both dermis and epidermis gradually thin, sweating ability is reduced and skin becomes more dry and fragile[5].

5 Waller, Jeanette M., and Howard I. Maibach. 'Age and Skin Structure and Function, a Quantitative Approach (I): ...'. *Skin Res. & Technol.*: ... 11, no. 4: 221–35

Layers of the skin

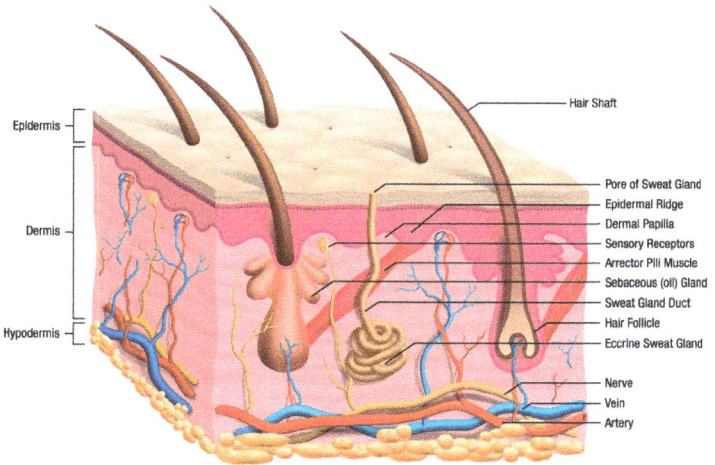

Epidermis – outer layer
Dermis – second layer
Subcutaneous – fatty layer

Absorption into the skin and tissues varies. Routes into the tissues go via:

- Intracellular
- Intercellular
- Through hair follicle roots
- Through sweat pores

Dermal absorption

Oils and fatty molecules are able to sink through the upper layers of the skin, water simply swells the outer skin cells (which causes wrinkly fingers in the bath). The combination of oils and waters in a cream have the best absorption rates as the molecules help each other pass through membranes. Below the top layers of skin the tissue chemistry changes and watery constituents within a cream can cross the lipid bilayer dissolving and absorbing deeper[6]. Smaller sized molecules will absorb more easily than large, and some constituents are able to pass through the capillaries into the bloodstream. This is how topical medications work, often applied by stick on patches. Some conditions and methods will enhance absorption.

- Covering the area such as patches or plasters
- Inclusion of ingredients such as alcohol
- Damp skin (such as after bathing)
- Warm skin (pores are open)
- Damaged skin absorbs more easily (beware when using potentially irritating products)
- Different areas of the body such as the face and inside of arms absorb well, thicker skinned areas are slower such as palms of the hands.

Some chemical additives such as sodium lauryl sulphate may appear to improve the feel of creams and soften

6 Carpentieri-Rodrigues et.al, 'Percutaneous Absorption Enhancers: Mechanisms and Potential'. *Brazil Arch. Biol. & Technol.* 50, no. 6: 949–61

the skin, however, they can irritate and dry the lower skin layers, ultimately creating dry and damaged skin[7].

Preservation

The following natural extracts are not preservatives in the strictest sense, however, they can be used to extend the life of your cream, and help to create a hostile environment to pathogens. Most bacteria and fungi require a fairly narrow range of optimum survival conditions to thrive. Much like we require food, water, comfortable temperature conditions and shelter, so do microbes. Creams have a high water content meaning spoilage is a higher risk. Disrupt the life cycle or conditions of microbes and this will help. Some additives attack the membrane 'bubble' surrounding certain types of bacteria, some reduce the ability to gain food or moisture, and some directly inhibit growth. It's worth knowing that manufactured natural preservatives usually have an optimum pH in which they are most effective, so check the descriptions when buying.

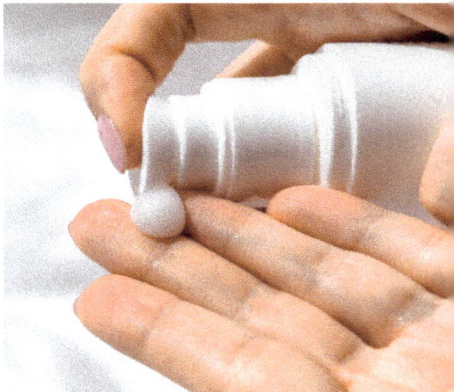

7 Burlando, Bruno et.al., *Herbal Principles in Cosmetics: Properties and Mechanisms of Action*. CRC Press, 2010.

Water solubles

● Grapefruit seed extract – a controversial ingredient which is sometimes said to be contaminated with things such as triclosan which is a chemical antibacterial, antifungal agent. However, an organic grapefruit seed extract is shown to be safe and can disrupt the bacterial membrane and slow pathogenic growth of some bacteria and mould[8].

● Alcohol – some addition of alcohol plant extracts or tinctures will inhibit growth of pathogens by attacking the bacterial membrane, small amounts in a cream are not drying to the skin, and can help add herb extracts to your cream.

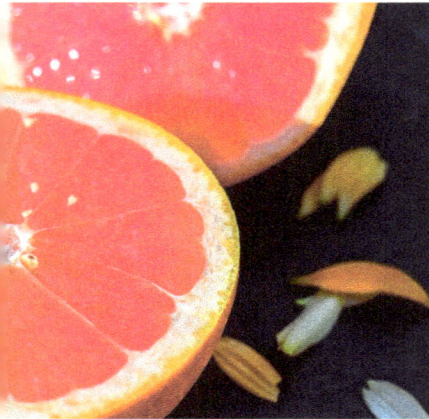

● Citric acid – usually available in a granular or powder form, a tiny amount added to the water phase of your cream making will control the pH balance helping make a hostile environment for pathogens. Originally made from citrus fruits but now commercially made by a fermentation process.

• Vegetable glycerine – an extract of fats from separation of fatty acids and glycerol which slows bacterial growth, can be drying in high amounts on the skin as it draws moisture from internal and external surroundings which is how it inhibits bacteria, however, in small amounts it is a useful moisturising addition which can also be used to extract botanical constituents[9].

Fat solubles

Oils and fats are slower to spoil than waters.

Oils and fats will ultimately turn rancid from oxygenation and free radical activity; this will be obvious by the smell. This can take weeks or months or years depending on the type of oil or fat, and how it has been processed and stored. Oils with a high polyunsaturated fatty acid content are the quickest to spoil, oils with a high level of monounsaturates last longer before going rancid, and those solid at room temperature in the northern hemisphere such as coconut, cocoa butter, and shea butter have the longest shelf life. Oxygenation and free radical activity can be slowed down by the addition of some natural extracts into your recipe.

• Vitamin E - either pure extract, or a little wheatgerm oil contains high levels of this vitamin[10].
• Rosemary antioxidant - an extract which is not an essential oil, and closer to a CO_2 extract, used in food

9 Chemistry Stack Exchange. 'Solutions - Does Glycerin Promote Bacterial Growth the Same as Water?'
10 The Dermatology Review. 'Should You Use a Vitamin E Cream?'.https://thedermreview.com/vitamin-e-cream/.

manufacturing and cosmetics for its effective inhibition of free radical formation[11].

Manufactured preservatives

This is by no means an exhaustive list, these are the ones I've tried and found effective and are of natural origin though manufactured in a lab. Extraction from their original source is unlikely to be achievable at home. Some brands combine two or more components to get a broad spectrum preservation and combat gram positive, gram negative bacteria, moulds and yeasts. If you aren't making your creams fresh for immediate use, you should use a preservative, and all bought in base creams will be using some type of preservative.

● Benzyl alcohol (and related benzoic acid and its salts, and benzyl benzoate) - can be of natural extract. Used in preparations to kill head lice. Potential allergen.
● Salicylic acid - found naturally in willow, meadowsweet and wintergreen and used as pain relief, can be of natural extract. Potential allergen.
● Potassium sorbate - can be of natural extract for instance from Rowan berries. Used in food preservation (such as supermarket hummus). Potential allergen.
● Gluconolactone - an antioxidant extracted by enzyme action of seed oils.

Allergens

11 Nieto, Gema, Gaspar Ros, and Julián Castillo. 'Antioxidant and Antimicrobial Properties of Rosemary (Rosmarinus Officinalis, L.): A Review'. *Medicines* 5, no. 3.

We are all different, and some people will react to natural ingredients the same as some react to synthetic ingredients. Concentrated extracts by their very nature are more likely to produce allergic reactions because of their strength. The European Commission lists 26 constituents which by law must be listed on a label if you are selling to the public. If you are making creams for your own use, friends, family or patients you should be aware of them and not exceed recommended manufacturer amounts, and suggest patch testing[12].

There are also recommended dermal limits on essential oils and other ingredients. There will be a manufacturer's safety data sheet with purchased ingredients. You may need to request this from the supplier, although some are available on the supplier websites automatically.

12 Introduction - European Commission' Perfume Allergies - Introduction.
https://ec.europa.eu/health/scientific_committees/opinions_layman/
perfume-allergies/en/index.htm

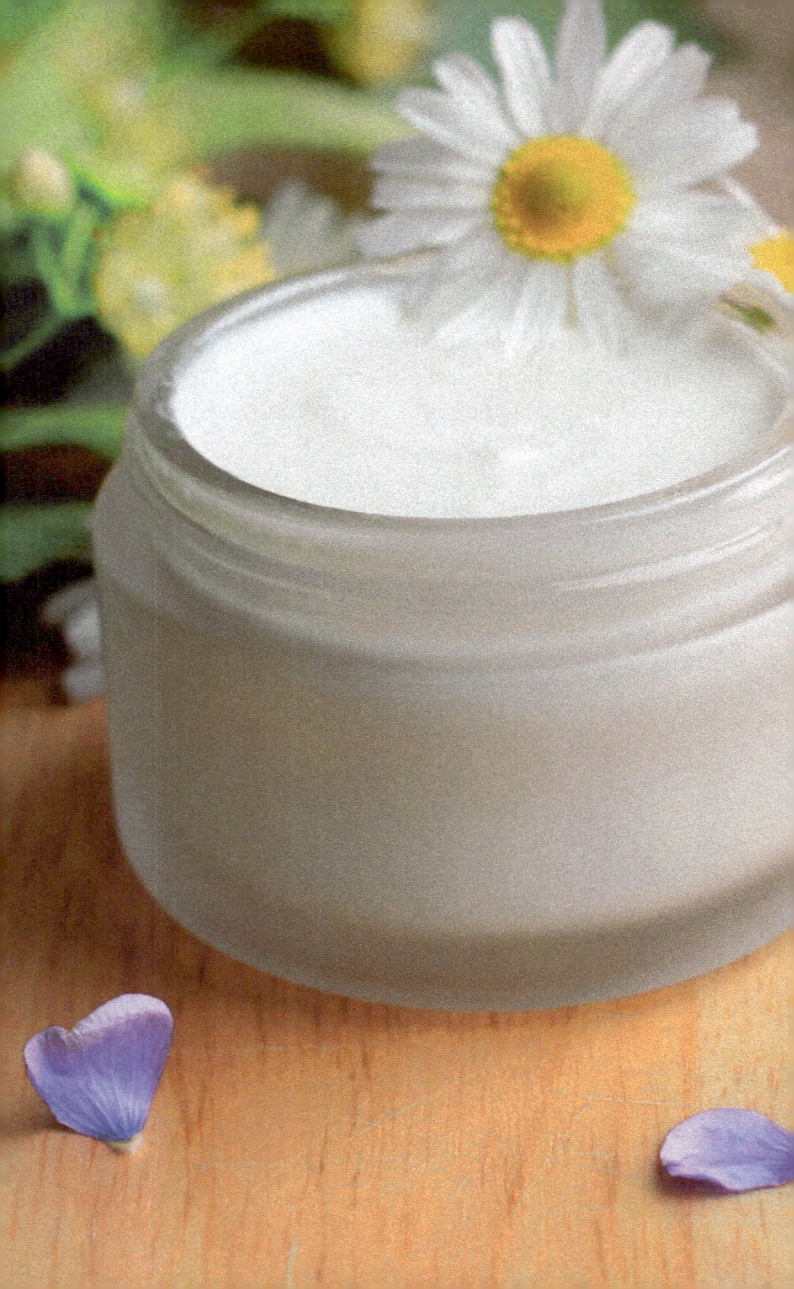

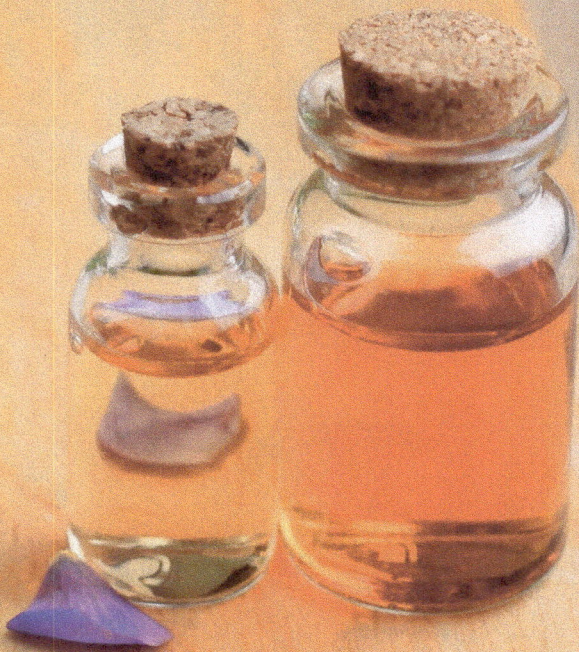

What makes a cream?

Building layers of botanicals for the most effective product

When making a cream or ointment for a patient I want it to be the most powerful it can be to combat their skin condition, and try to get the herbs into the product that will work synergistically with each other, enhancing the efficacy. You are unlikely to get this from a commercially manufactured product.

This can be done by including any or all of the following:

- Hydrosols
- Teas
- Glycerites
- Macerated oils
- Tinctures
- Fresh plant juice
- Essential oils
- CO_2 extracts
- Macerated solid fats

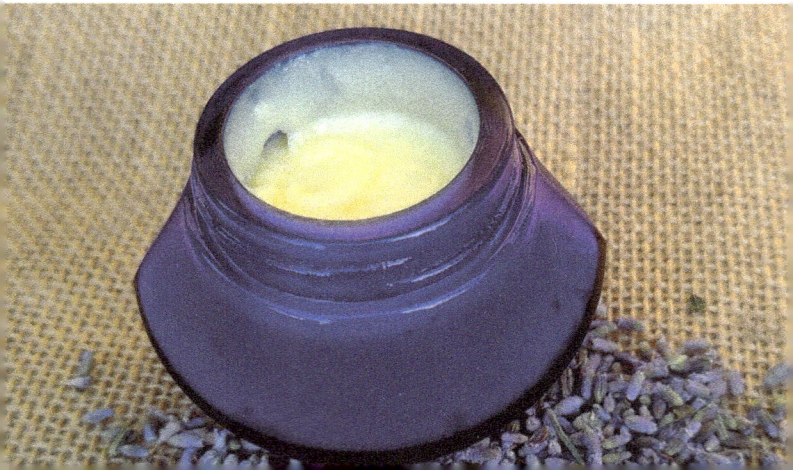

Hydrosols

These are sometimes called hydrolats, or floral waters. If you are buying them, ensure they are distilled extracts, not water with essential oil and a chemical dispersant.

They may or may not have preservative. If unpreserved you will need to either buy in small amounts and refrigerate, or add your own preservative, or they can be frozen and defrosted in small amounts for immediate use. Though some people prefer not to freeze as they feel the product is damaged much like you know a vegetable is not the same when it's been frozen as it was fresh.

A hydrosol will last a lot longer than a tea, follow the label best before dates, they usually last unopened for several months. Once open keep chilled and follow the label instructions about how long it lasts after opening, this is an open lid jar symbol with a number and the letter M such as 6M for 6 months. If you are lucky enough to have your own still and make your own hydrosols, you can either add preservative, freeze, or keep chilled. A useful tip that helps to know if the hydrosol is ok apart from the appearance and smell, is to check the pH the day after making it, note it and the date, and check every month thereafter. If the pH starts to rise, become more alkaline, there is likely to be some sort of bacterial or fungal spoilage.

Hydrosols add a wonderful dimension to creams rather than using plain water, the lighter molecules such as esters and some volatile oils are present adding to the fragrance and the healing properties.

Not everybody has a still of course. I attended a wonderful talk by Rosemary Gladstar, the lovely American herbalist, who has written many books. She described a practical way to make a hydrosol using just your kitchen equipment. I have tried this, and made a comparison alongside using a still with the same herb, fennel seed. The comparison was good, the still extract was stronger, but the other was a good second, and perfectly useable.

You need a large pan with a domed lid. Two heat proof bowls which easily stack back to back inside the pan with plenty of room.

Place one bowl upside down in the pan, and fill with water just up to the base, leaving a centimeter or so clear out of the water. Add some chopped herb material and push under the water. Place your second

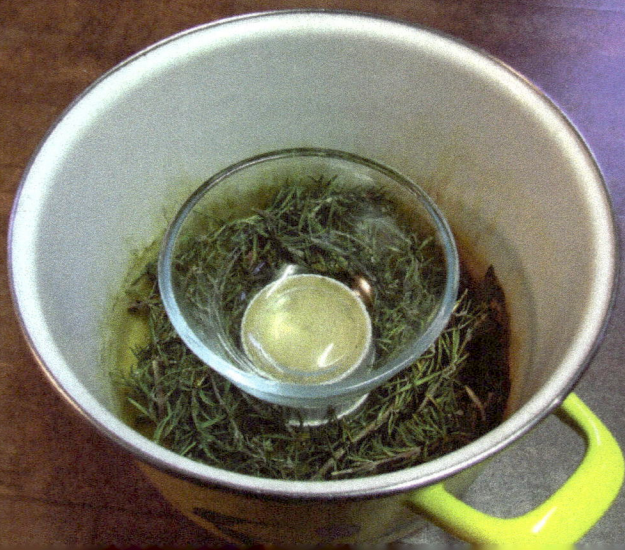

heat proof bowl ontop of the first, upright. This will be your collection bowl for the hydrosol. Place your lid onto your pan upside down, so the domed part faces down inside the pan. Place the pan on the heat and gently bring to a simmer, without getting to a fierce boil. If you have ice packs, place some in the lid of the pan, or if not, cold water will work. This will need to be regularly changed, so it helps if you have it contained in a bag of some sort.

As the herb scented steam rises and hits the cold pan lid, it forms condensation which rolls down the dome shape of the lid and drips into the catchment bowl. If you have a see through domed pan lid this is perfect as you can keep an eye on it without losing steam by opening it up. Before the pan boils dry, remove from the heat and allow to cool. The hydrosol should be stored in a bottle out of the light, and preferably at cool temperatures. You can add 10% alcohol to help preserve if required.

Teas

A simple herb or flower tea in place of the water portion of a cream adds to the healing ingredients, and should be made fresh and used immediately. Efficient straining with a fine mesh strainer or muslin cloth is important to avoid plant particles increasing mould or bacterial contamination risk.

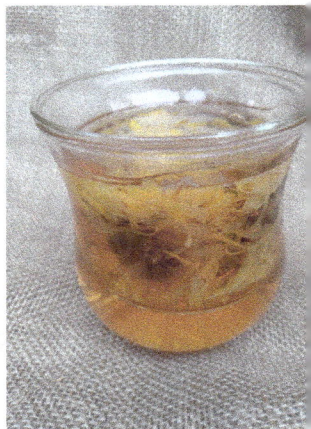

Glycerites

These are a useful way to add plant power to a cream and aid the moisturising effect when used at small amounts, up to 5%. There is no right or wrong way to make a glycerite, a macerated glycerine extract. You can buy a few from herb suppliers, such as chamomile or rose, but they are easy to make.

These are my favourite ways to prepare them and they should keep for a year.

- Macerate plant matter, fresh or dried in a mix of 60% glycerine and 40% water for a couple of weeks, strain and keep for future use.
- Juice fresh plant material (only works well with sap-rich plants, for instance plantain or cleavers) use the juice at 40% and blend with 60% of vegetable glycerine.
- Make a strong tea infusion, strain and mix at 40% to 60% vegetable glycerine.

Macerated oils

There are a couple of ways to do this, using fresh or dried plant material, the hot or cold methods, and everyone will have their favoured way. Pack your clean and dry plant matter (fresh dry as in no dew or rain on the plant, or dried plant) into a jar, and cover with your preferred vegetable oil making sure the plant material stays underneath the surface. You can use a clean pebble, or glass 'pickle pebble' to ensure this, or a smaller empty jar to push it down.

• Hot method: Place the jar in a pan or slow cooker of water reaching halfway up your jar. Warm gently for several hours, or overnight in the slow cooker, ensuring water levels don't drop. Remove; dry the outside of the jar and strain off your oil, store in a dark cupboard.

• Cold method (sometimes called the sun method, or even the moonlight method): Ensuring your plant matter stays below the surface of the oil to avoid moulding, place your jar, covered with a muslin dust cloth, on a sunny windowsill to breakdown in the sun and or moonlight. This works well with Hypericum, which is traditionally called a sunshine herb.

Tinctures

The various methods and measurements are beyond the scope of this book and need an alcohol licence to purchase the 96% high strength spirit. However, tinctures are easily available to buy ready-made, or you can use vodka which will be an all-round strength suitable for most herbs. Make tinctures by soaking plant material in neat vodka, keeping plant material underneath the surface, shaking daily. Strain after 2 - 6 weeks or so, and keep out of sunlight once made. This will keep for at least two years for most herbs. Follow the recipes and limit the amount of tincture, high amounts can be

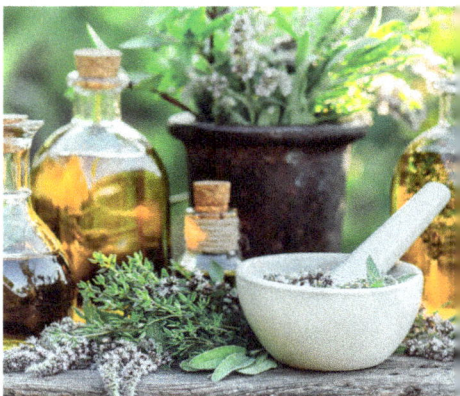

irritating and drying to the skin, but also may prevent your cream from blending properly.

Fresh Plant Juice

Easiest to make using a blender or juicer, though certain herbs can be crushed and squeezed by hand when fresh, such as chickweed. These make a powerful addition to a cream, though are likely to spoil quickly, and should be stored in the fridge, or a preservative method used. This would form part of your water portion, so reduce the hydrosol, tea or water by about 10% and replace with the juice.

Essential oils

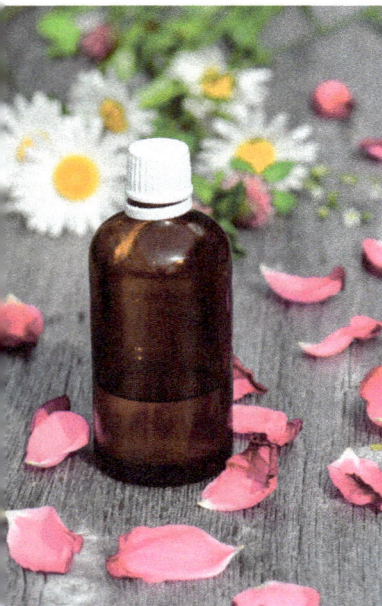

I am not an aromatherapist. Most essential oils are too strong to be used neat on the skin, however, with some it is possible such as lavender, do your own research on this. Check my bibliography for books on essential oils. As delicate and volatile substances, these should be treated with great respect and not wasted. A huge amount of plant matter is used to make tiny amounts of oil and as with any precious material, should be used mindfully. There are different ways of extracting the oils, some using chemical extraction, some steam distilled, some water distilled and some cold pressed such as for the citrus oils. The healing benefits are not just from application to the skin, but from the fragrance breathed in which travels directly to the limbic system in the brain. Depending on the oil, I use an average of 10 drops per 60ml pot of cream. Some medicinal effects need higher doses but the recommended dermal limits should be followed. Oils such as Gaultheria procumbens (Wintergreen) used for pain relief need careful consideration. *The European Directorate for the Quality of Medicines & HealthCare* has some useful information under their essential oils section. Some oils such as citrus oils increase the sensitivity of the skin to sunlight exposure. The *Aromatherapy Trade Council* has some useful links and safety information, though it is worth noting that this refers to cosmetic products, whereas when needing medicinal benefits, more may be needed[13].

CO_2 extracts

These are plant extracts created by use of CO_2. They are pure extracts and organic is available too. They should be used in a similar way to essential oils, as they are just as potent but will have a wider range of constituents from the plant including the heavier molecules such as tannins. The temperatures needed for extraction are lower than those used in distillation, which can be of

13 'Essential Oil Safety : Aromatherapy Trade Council'. https://www.a-t-c. org.uk/safety-matters/essential-oil-safety/

benefit though the fragrance is not usually as powerful as essential oils[14].

Macerated solid fats

On the theme of packing as many herbs into your healing product as possible, you can macerate, or soak solid fats with herbs too. In a cool climate such as the U.K. coconut oil, cocoa butter, shea butter and most waxes will remain solid at room temperature. You can use a gentle warming plate overnight, or a bowl in a slow cooker placed in a water bath. This keeps the solid fat in a liquid state in order to extract some plant constituents, strain off and then store the fat, carefully labelled. I have found this to work very well with coconut oil, cocoa butter and shea butter.

Fixed or Carrier oils

Your choice of oils is governed by the therapeutic aim, the compliance of use, (such as avoiding very sticky or heavy oils for those who need a quick absorbing light cream) and affordability. Oils such as cold pressed rosehip and jojoba cost several times more per litre than sunflower or olive oils, especially if organic. In this case it's useful to blend two or more together to gain the therapeutic benefit balanced with affordability.

Most oils will have their own therapeutic benefit to add to a cream. For the purposes of this guide the term oils means those products that are liquid at room

14 Díaz-Maroto, M.et;al,. 'Supercritical Carbon Dioxide Extraction of Volatiles from Spices: Comparison with Simultaneous Distillation–Extraction'. *Journal of Chromatography* A 947, no. 1: 23–29.

temperature all year round in the UK. The following list of oils is not exhaustive but a few examples of those I use, see the bibliography at the end for further reading.

Fixed or carrier oils can be used with or without added herbal maceration. Care should be taken to check plant origins if treating someone with allergies for example nut allergies. Gluten proteins should not be present in the oil, and in any case are said to be too large for topical absorption. However, someone who is coeliac or even gluten intolerant may find they have a general sensitivity to wheatgerm oil itself, including on the skin, so an alternative may be sensible.

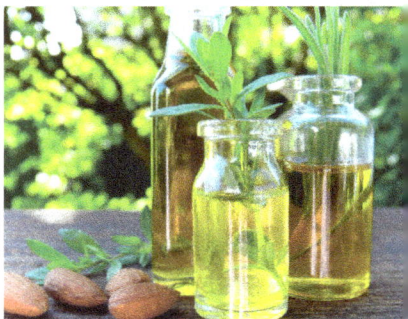

- Almond oil (*Amygdalus communis*): a rich nourishing nut oil high in vitamin E with a good shelf life

- Avocado oil (*Persea gratissima*): pressed from the flesh of the avocado pear, this oil contains carotenoids, B vitamins and vitamin E. Forms a light protective barrier with anti-inflammatory properties.

- Castor Bean oil (*Ricinus communis*): a very thick, sticky oil not therefore not often used in creams, but with a therapeutic benefit in castor oil skin packs for pain relief and constipation

- Grape Seed oil (*Vitis vinifera*): pressed from the seeds of grapes after the juice is extracted. A medium rich oil, easily absorbed, containing good levels of vitamin E and proanthocyanadins which support collagen and elastin.

- Jojoba oil (Simmondsia chinensis): technically a liquid

wax which will solidify if refrigerated. One of the best absorbed oils through the layers of the skin with high ability to protect against drying, without blocking pores, so a good one to include for dry skin conditions such as eczema. This oil has a very long shelf life.

● Olive Oil (Olea europaea): a medium-rich fragrant oil which some people enjoy and others dislike, which is something to take into account. High in squalene which is a natural sebum constituent of the skin. Healing after sun exposure.

● Rosehip Seed oil (Rosa rubiginosa): extracted from the rosehip seeds, cold pressed is best. Very rich in vitamin E and carotenoids, rosehip oil is of benefit for reducing scarring and promoting healing.

● Sunflower Oil (Helianthus annuus): a nourishing oil with good amounts of vitamin E. This oil has a short shelf life and is best bought in small amounts and used quickly.

● Wheatgerm oil (Triticum vulgare): very rich in vitamin E and improves microcirculation.

Fats and butters which are solid at room temperature (Northern hemisphere)

● Cocoa Butter (*Theobroma cacao*): everyone knows this popular fat, used in chocolate making. Melts at body temperature, this makes cocoa butter very useful for making pessaries and suppositories, and it is a rich emollient addition to a cream forming a light protective barrier. Also useful in salves for this purpose.

● Coconut Oil (*Cocos nucifera*): useful in salves for its soft oily texture, coconut oil is naturally anti-inflammatory and has some anti-fungal and anti-bacterial properties. The melting temperature is 25°C.

• Shea butter (*Butyrospermum parkii*): a solid yet soft fat which forms a thin protective layer on the skin. Can be used for enfleurage, the extraction of essential oils from delicate flowers such as ylang ylang and neroli by spreading a layer of fat, covered with flowers, then another layer of fat pressed between two plates of glass. The melting temperature is 70°C.

Note that often a fat may appear melted, but until you reach the listed temperature you may find some fatty acids are actually still solid, and that will mean a grainy resulting cream.
You can purchase many oil waxes and butters processed from oils such as Almond and Sunflower, often these are created by hydrogenation, adding hydrogen and creating trans-fats, and you can decide whether you

Image below. Bottom left clockwise: coconut fat, shea butter, cocoa butter, carnauba wax and centre candelilla wax

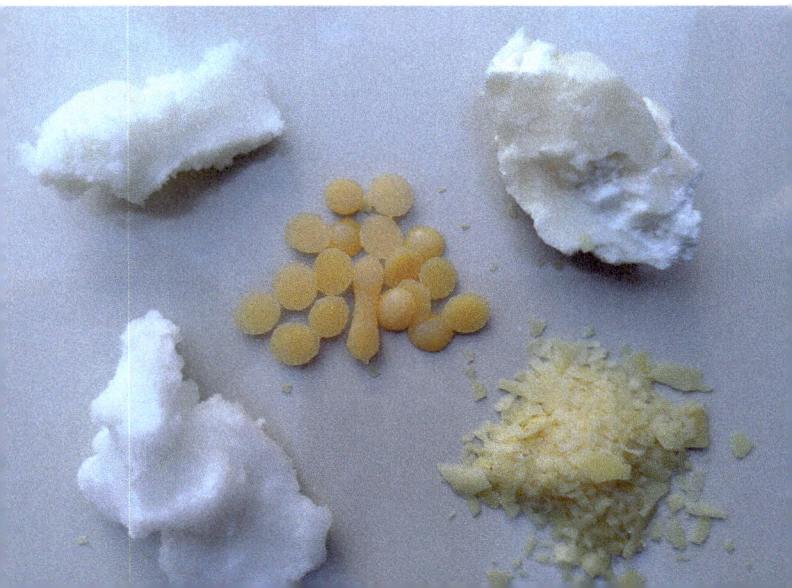

want to use these depending on how natural you want your cream to be. These would be used in place of the above fats in a recipe. Similarly palm fat could be used, and if you decide to use this please choose from ethically produced and grown sources.

Plant Waxes

These are fats, usually sold in pellet form, which remain solid even in warm temperatures, and need heat to melt down. They can have a slight emulsifying effect, and are used in low amounts to add protective properties to a cream. Listed below are a few I've used.

- Bayberry wax (*Myrica cerifera*): a pale green wax with a pleasant aroma, this is obtained by boiling the berries from the Wax Myrtle shrub grown commonly in the USA and Columbia. The melting temperature is approximately 50°C.
- Candelilla wax (*Euphorbia cerifera*): sold in yellow hard pellets, this is obtained by heat extraction from the leaves of the Candelilla shrub, native to Mexico and South America. It has a melting temperature of 72°C, so when using in a cream you need to melt both the water phase and the oil phase to this temperature.
- Carnauba wax (*Copernicia cerifera*): this wax is removed by pounding the leaves. It is grown in Brazil. It has a very high melting temperature of 82°C which is an advantage when you want a very hard stable product, such as lip balms, but a disadvantage when you prefer not to heat other ingredients to such a high temperature such as unstable delicate oils like sunflower which is high in polyunsaturated fatty acids.

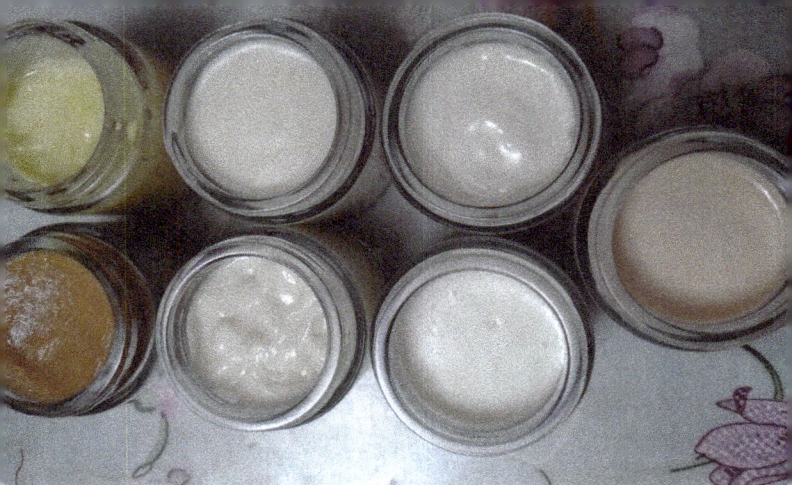

Image above. Clockwise from top left: whipped balm, medium cream, light cream, lecithin lotion, mousse lotion, thick cream, ointment salve.

Emulsifiers

As mentioned in the introduction, the inclusion of an emulsifier will make a stable, smooth product which keeps its integrity even at different environmental temperatures. Without this you may get separation of different fatty acids melting at various temperatures, leading to a gritty or granular salve, or a separated cream with increased risk of spoilage. Having said that, I do have a whipped butter recipe which uses a method of whip and cool and repeat until a fairly stable buttery consistency product is obtained. In extremely hot conditions this does soften but should retain its smooth texture.

Many emulsifiers are synthetic, but the following list are just a few I have tried and found effective. They are created in a lab setting, but made from natural components.

Some emulsify but don't thicken, so you get a thin but blended lotion type consistency, some thicken and emulsify together. Often you may need an emulsifier and a thickener to obtain the best result. Experiment, but always make notes as you need to recreate that perfect cream once achieved.

The term alcohol is a chemistry classification and not related to the fermented alcohol consumed as a drink.

● Cetearyl alcohol: Cetearyl alcohol is a fatty triglyceride, a blend of cetyl and stearyl alcohol which gives stability and is a thickener as well as emulsifier.
● Cetearyl alcohol and cetearyl glucoside (also known as Vegetal): when you melt vegetal the emulsifying bonds separate. As you initially whisk fast on blending they join and attach to each other for the first minute, after that you run the risk of them breaking apart again if you whisk too fast. So one minute to blend quickly, then slow stirring to maintain the smooth consistency. Added to the oils stage.
● Cetyl alcohol: this is more of a thickener than just an emulsifier, and needs a co-emulsifier to work. Helps create a smooth custard type consistency.
● Coco glucoside: classified chemically as a natural surfactant, working in the same way as an emulsifier, which means it emulsifies but can also be used in a cream to make a mousse style light non greasy cream when used with a thickener. Added to the water stage.
● Glyceryl stearate citrate: a very gentle emulsifier. It has the consistency of syrup and is used as a co-emulsifier alongside thickeners. Added to the oils stage.
● Glyceryl stearate: classed as a co-emulsifier this

creates a silky, non-greasy stable product but may need a thickening emulsifier if you want a consistency more than a thin lotion. A benefit of this product is it helps you include quite heavy oils such as castor oil and keeps the consistency non greasy. Added to the oils stage.

● Lecithin: the most natural emulsifier, usually extracted from sunflower seeds or soya beans. It comes in a syrup type form, and is a dark brown colour, so this does influence the final colour of your product. However, in a cream or lotion, the colour is creamy yellow.

Image below. Bottom left clockwise: Glyceryl Stearate, Lecithin, Coco Glucoside, Vegetal, Cetyl Alcohol, Candelilla Wax and centre Cetearyl Alcohol.

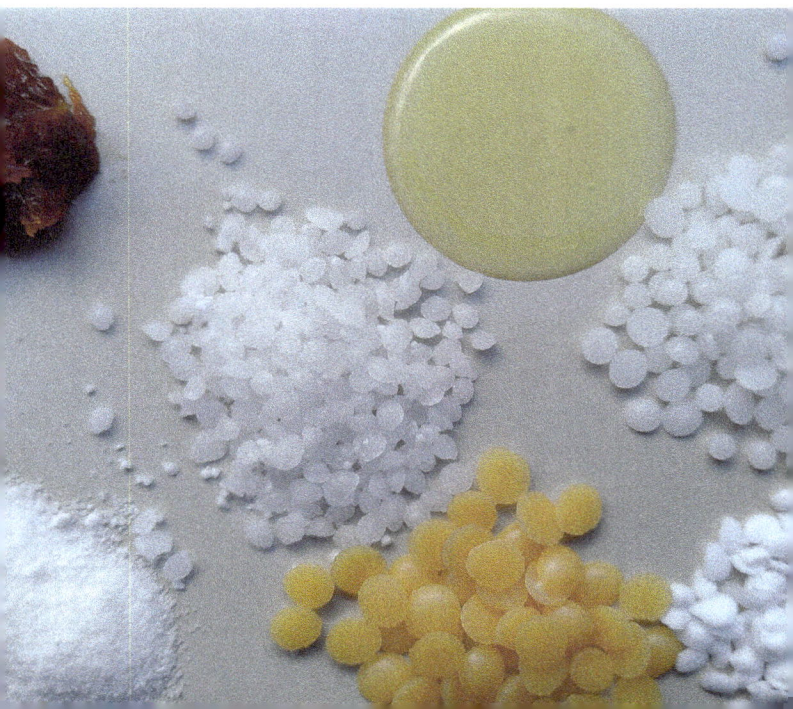

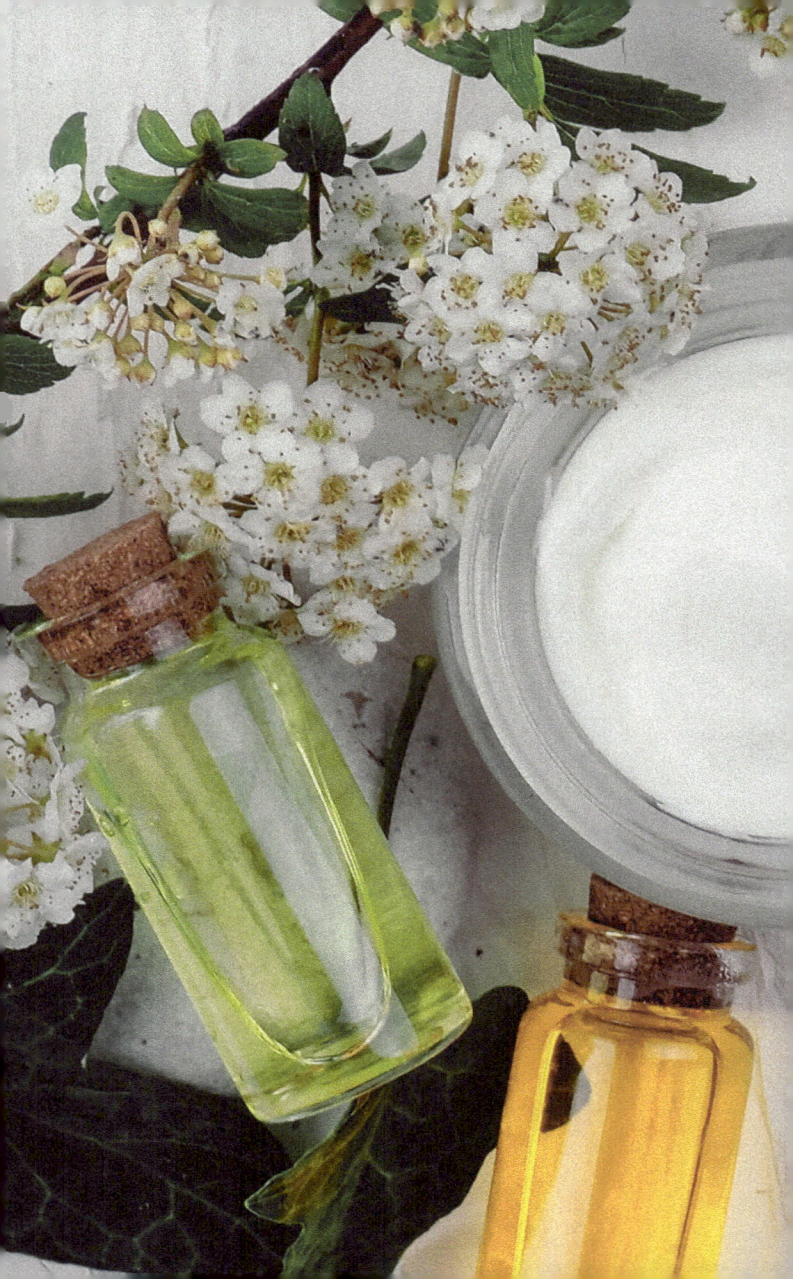

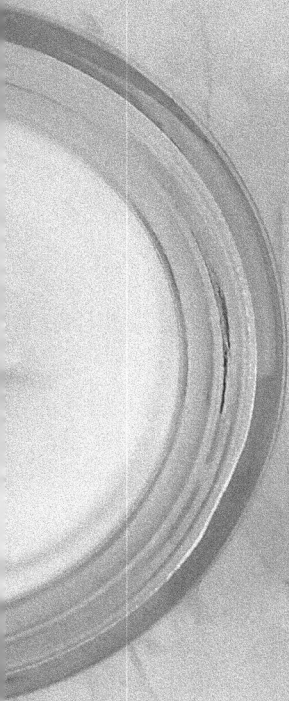

Skin care herbs

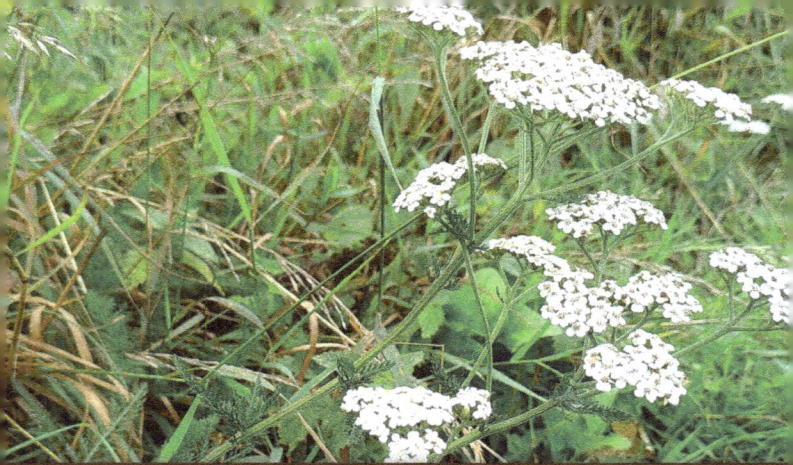

Yarrow
Achillea millefolium

This herb has an ancient tradition of being used to heal wounds backed up by modern use[15]. The volatile oils are antiseptic, and the tannins amongst other constituents promote healing and new healthy skin cell regeneration. The leaves and or flowers are used and can be made into a skin wash, poultice, macerated (steeped in any vegetable carrier oil) oils or made into tincture to include in a cream. The essential oil is commercially available, and is dark blue due to the azulene content, similar to Chamomilla recutitia. The essential oil is anti-inflammatory, antiseptic and in human volunteers showed a beneficial result in comparison with a mild hydrocortisone cream[16].

15 Hajashami et. al., *The effect of Achillea millefolium and Hypericum perforatum ointments on episiotomy wound healing in primiparous women*
16 Guarrera, M., et.al., 'The Anti-Inflammatory Activity of Azulene'. *J. Eur. Ac. Derm & Ven*. 15, no. 5: 486–87

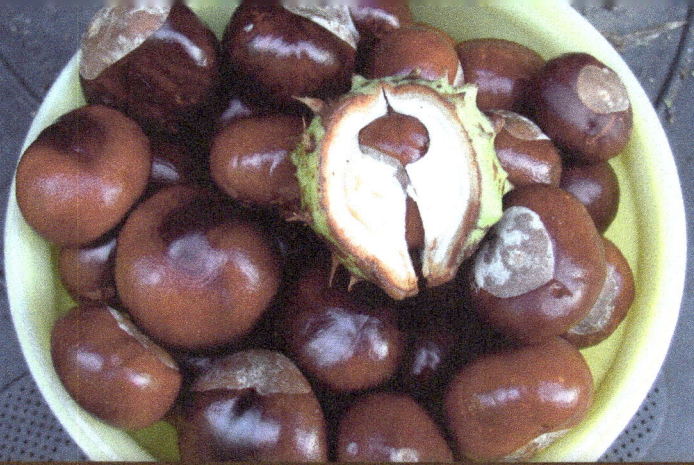

Horse chestnut/conker
Aesculus hippocastanum

The brown shiny conkers much loved by children are an effective herbal remedy for combatting venous insufficiency and capillary fragility. In fact research shows the flowers are also useful in wound healing[17].

They are harvested as they fall from the trees, discarding the prickly green shell, and chopping the inner conker whilst fresh. Once it's dried they are impossible to chop up. (Unless you use a garden shredder!)

They can be tinctured for use in a cream; the main medicinal constituents are water soluble saponins, and tannins. They could also be decocted (boiled) in water for immediate use as the water portion in a cream.

17 Suter, A, et.al., 'Treatment of Patients with Venous Insufficiency with Fresh Plant Horse Chestnut Seed Extract: A Review of 5 Clinical Studies'. *Advances in Therapy* 23, no. 1: 179–90

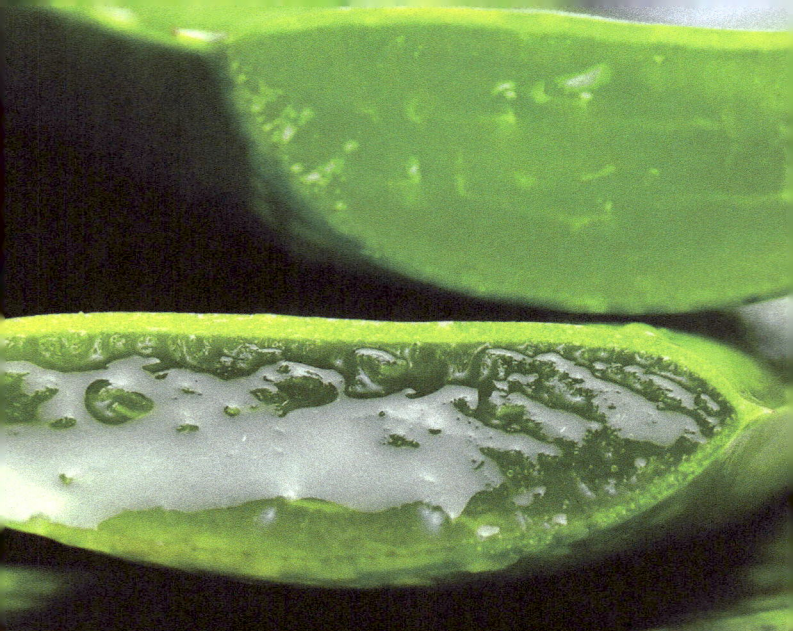

Aloe Vera
Aloe vera

A ready-made skin soothing healer, every kitchen should have a few Aloe vera plants which grow very happily and proliferate in most cases. The thick gel inside the leaves is an instant relief for minor burns, including sunburn and grazes. I find it quite fiddly to extract larger amounts from the leaves in a usable form to mash and add other ingredients. The easiest method I have found is to freeze a few leaves, then the gel is more easily removed. Bought ready-made gel is a quick easy option to which you can add 10-20% tinctures, and essential oils.

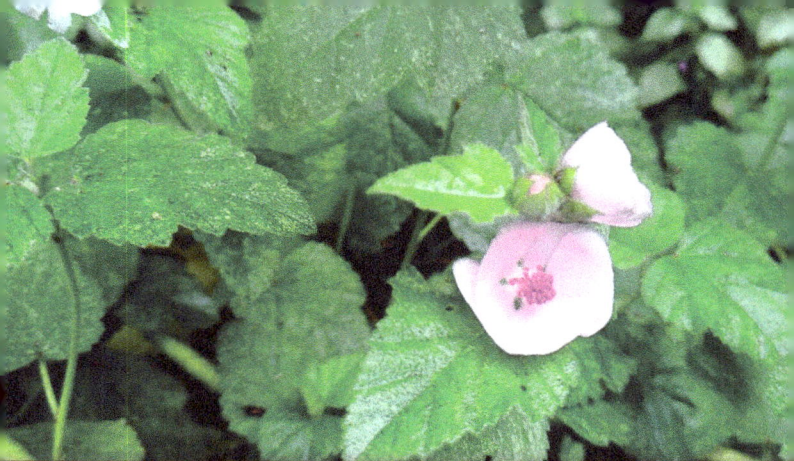

Marshmallow
Althaea officinalis

The roots and leaves of this soothing, anti-inflammatory plant are of great benefit for easing irritations and sore skin. A poultice can also be made as a drawing paste to pull out small splinters, and to draw pus from wounds. The more common mallow Malva sylvestris, the tree mallow Lavetera maritima and others are usable in the same way if you have no access to Marshmallow. The closest in the strength of relevant constituents to Marshmallow is the Tree Mallow.

The polysaccharides in the mallow family form a gel like layer on the skin offering protection and reducing irritations whatever the cause. I often use this as one of many herbs in creams for psoriasis or eczema when the dry heat in the skin needs cooling and moistening[18].

18 Bonaterra,G.A,. 'Anti-Inflammatory and Anti-Oxidative Effects of Phytohustil® and Root Extract of Althaea Officinalis L. on Macrophages in Vitro'. *Frontiers in Pharmacology* 11.

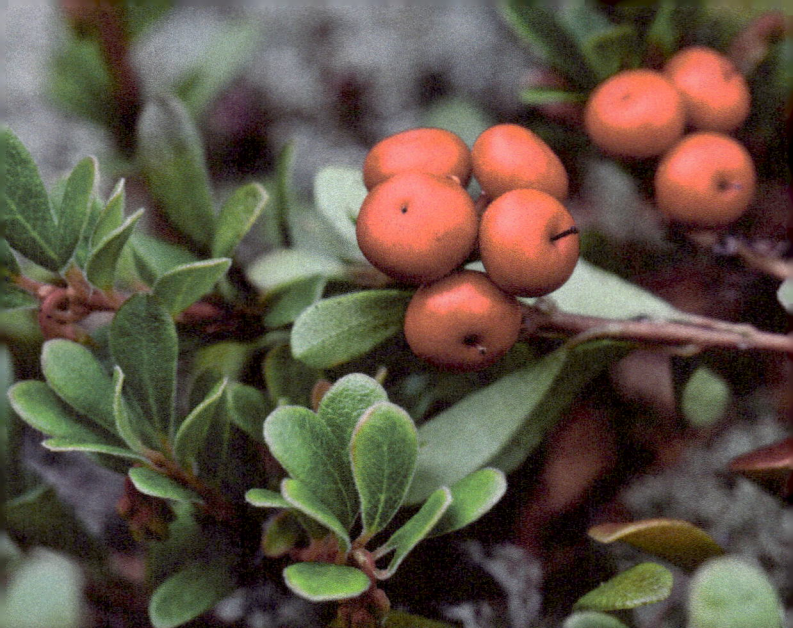

Bearberry
Arctostaphylos uva-ursi

This herb is traditionally known for internal use orally treating cystitis, however, it's interesting to learn that externally it can be helpful for hyperpigmentation, dark patches on the skin which can be triggered by hormonal changes such as pregnancy, taking the contraceptive pill or menopause. Believed to be the arbutin constituent of Uva-ursi, an extract in a cream alongside phytoestrogenic herbs can be helpful[19].

19 American Academy of Dermatology. 'Natural ingredients used in new topical treatments for hyperpigmentation: Dermatologists explains.'

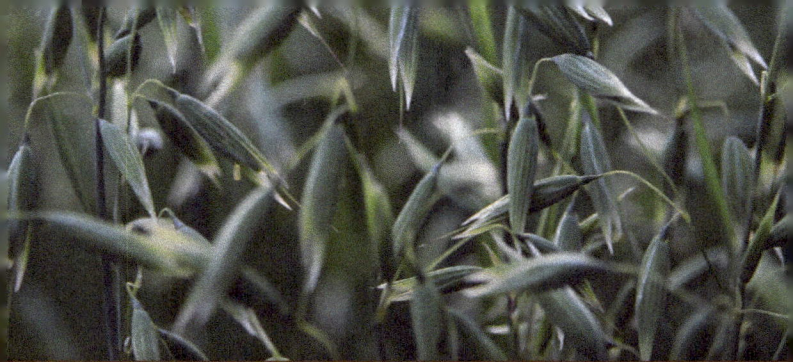

Oats
Avena sativa

Oats are well known for their anti-inflammatory action on the skin. Commonly used to help soothe eczema, (Grimalt, 2007) a handful of ordinary porridge oats in an old sock or tied in a square of muslin and swished about in a bath creates a soothing, milky fluid that reduces itching and inflammation. It is possible to include a cold infusion of oats in a cream as some of your hydrosol or tea portion, perhaps 50%, though I'd suggest doubling up on preservation as the polysaccharides are prone to going off quickly. You can also include approximately half a teaspoon of colloidal oatmeal (fine ground porridge oats powder, easy to make from porridge oats) to a cream, easier if blended with a teaspoon of glycerine first to avoid clumping.

An easier way is to include oat tincture, or to purchase Oat CO_2 extract and use a couple of drops blended into the finished cream. You can also purchase colloidal oat powder which is easy to use and has been shown to improve and maintain skin recovery in eczema[20].

20 Sobhan, M, 'The Efficacy of Colloidal Oatmeal Cream 1% as Add-on Therapy in the Management of Chronic Irritant Hand Eczema: A Double-Blind Study'. Clin. *Cos. & Inv. Derm*. 13 : 241–51

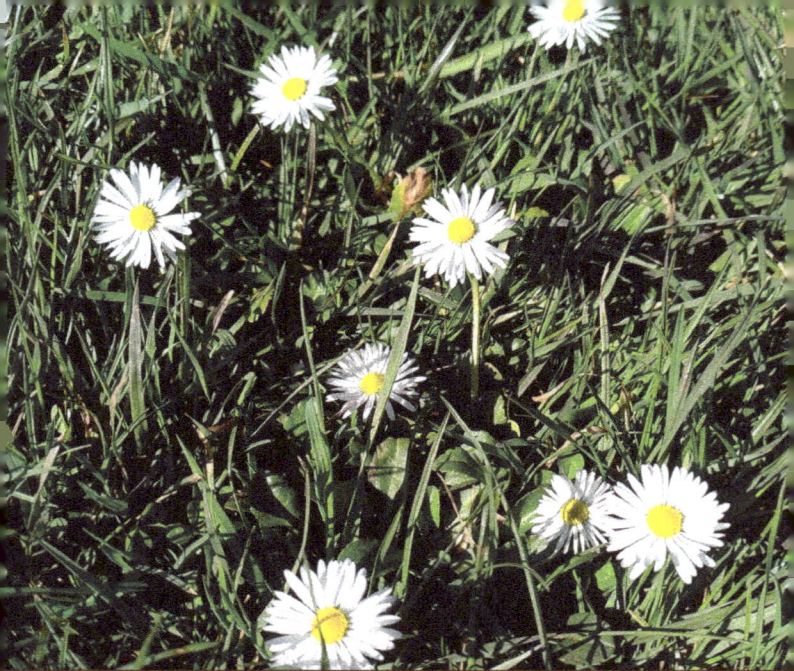

Daisy
Bellis perennis

Known in herbalists' circles in the UK as our native version of Arnica, the old country name of Bruisewort (wort meaning herb) describes the use of daisy flowers very well. The flowers and leaves are used, and can be made into tincture, dried or fresh. Oxeye Daisy flowers can also be used.

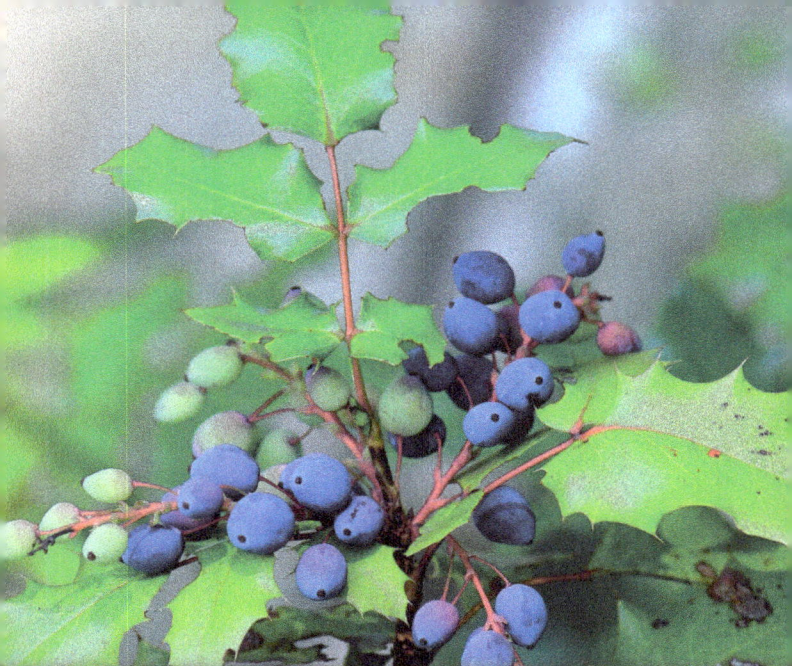

Barberry and Oregon Grape
Berberis vulgaris and *Berberis aquifolium*

Potent antibacterial action from the bark and root bark of these shrubs has been shown to have a good effect on reducing severity of psoriasis, helping reduce dryness and down regulate inflammatory responses in previously treatment resistant conditions[21]. In that study a herbal wash was used, I have used tincture blended into a cream with some success.

21 Brinker, F. 'Psoriasis Treatment with Oregon Grape Extracts'

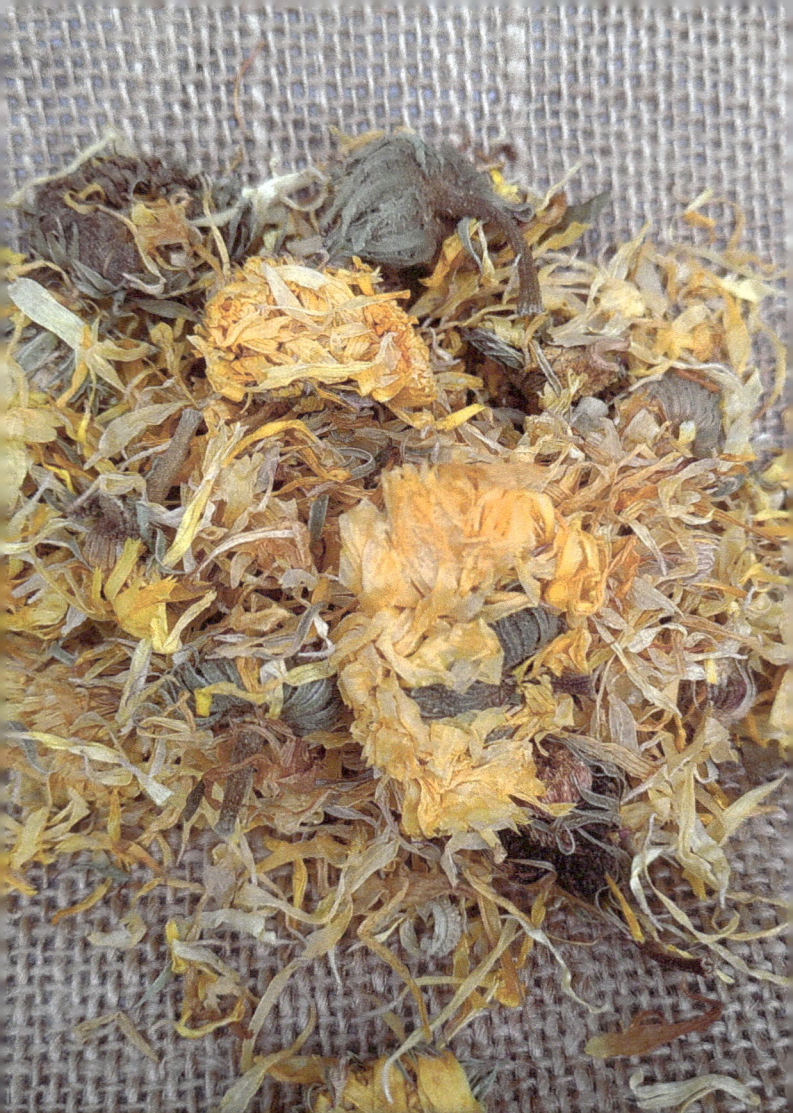

Pot marigold
Calendula officinalis

Bright orange, sometimes yellow flowers in the daisy family. The name originates because the flowers are present almost every calendar month of the year. Studies show the polysaccharides promote granulation of healthy new skin cells, therefore promoting and speeding up healing. There are also resins present which show anti-fungal and antiseptic action.

The flower heads can be macerated in a carrier oil, or used as a tea, hydrosol or tincture in creams. You can also purchase precious expensive essential oil, and CO_2 extracts for a very concentrated extract in a cream. The latter two items must be diluted and are only used at a drop or two per pot of approximately 60 ml cream.

There are two different actions from this glorious cheerful flower. The healing and anti-inflammatory action, flavonoids extracted by water or low alcohol tinctures, 25-45% alcohol to water ratio for example, and the terpenes and resins which are extracted with high alcohol tinctures of 90% alcohol content.

Studies show anti-inflammatory, healing promotion and anti-microbial action on gut walls, mouth, gums, and skin cells[22,23].

Both traditional herbal medicine and modern research supports the benefit of Calendula in speeding up the healing of wounds[24].

22 Colombo, E, et al., 'A Bio-Guided Fractionation to Assess the Inhibitory Activity of Calendula Officinalis L. on the NF-KB Driven Transcription in Human Gastric Epithelial Cells'. *ECAM* 2015 .
23 Saini, P. et al., 'Effects of Calendula Officinalis on Human Gingival Fibroblasts'. *Homeopathy: The Journal of the Faculty of Homeopathy* 101, no. 2:92–98
24 Nicolaus.,'*In Vitro Studies to Evaluate the Wound Healing Properties of Calendula Officinalis Extracts*'

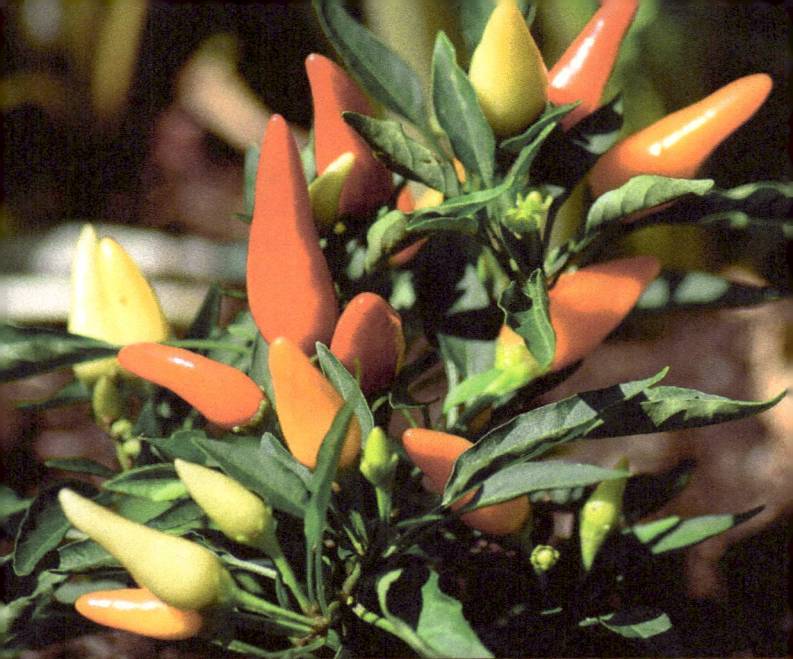

Chilli pepper
Capsicum spp.

A powerful addition to pain relieving products. All the chilli family have the heat producing constituents which we use in cooking. When applied (diluted in oil, or creams) in small amounts on the skin the effect is to interfere with the pain messaging neurotransmitters telling our brain we are in pain. This has shown to be effective for soft tissue pain, arthritic pain and nerve pain[25].

A small study on burning mouth syndrome showed benefits of pain relief using capsicum gel over a period of time[26].

It is important to note that the analgesic constituents within the plant material are lipophilic or fat soluble, so a water extract will be ineffective. Use a chilli tincture, or chilli oil in small amounts such as 5ml per 100ml of cream. Some skin warming or even irritation can occur, this is normal and unless severe, (in which case wash it off with soapy water), and part of the process. The counter irritant effects can also relieve pressure in swollen joints, the blood being pulled to the skin surface by the warmth, draws congested fluids from joints, gets the circulation moving again; improving the removal of toxic metabolites while helping to deliver nutrients.

It is also interesting to note that although the trend is to use capsicum for these benefits, similar benefits can be gained from use of mustard instead. Our own native wild mustard is easily available and the leaves can be used instead of the seeds.

A word of caution, all the above additions have the potential to cause burning and blistering of the skin, so small amounts, carefully tried out initially, especially for those with sensitive skin, and in the very young and elderly.

25 Frederick H. et.al., 'Topical Treatment of Chronic Low Back Pain with a Capsicum Plaster' *Pain* 106: 59–64.
26 Jørgensen, M, and Pedersen, A., 'Analgesic Effect of Topical Oral Capsaicin Gel in Burning Mouth Syndrome'. *Acta Odontologica Scandinavica* 75, no. 2: 130–36

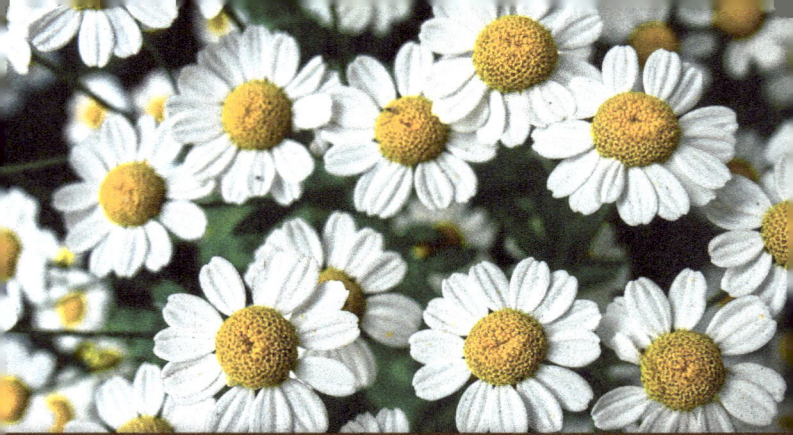

German and Roman chamomile
Matricaria/Chamomilla recutita & Anthemis nobilis

Well known for the calming benefits in a tea, chamomile is used in skin treatments for bringing down inflammation and soothing irritations. Used in the form of essential oils, water extracts, macerated in carrier oils or tinctures in cream making, the flowers of both types of chamomile are effective at calming irritations and skin inflammation whatever the cause may be. The absorption of the anti-inflammatory constituents is shown to reach deep layers of the skin[27].

The essential oil of the German Chamomile *(Matricaria* or *Chamomilla recutita*) is dark blue due to the azulene constituent, distillation of some types of wild yarrow also contain azulene and the essential oil is dark blue. Highly anti-inflammatory, both these oils are expensive and precious, to be used sparingly and wisely.

27 Merfort, I. et. al., 'In Vivo Skin Penetration Studies of Camomile Flavones'. *Die Pharmazie* 49, no. 7: 509–11.

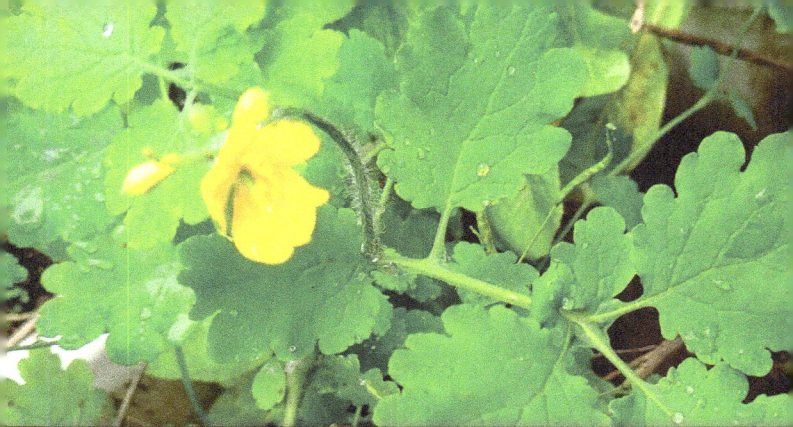

Greater celandine
Chelidonium majus

Greater Celandine is a restricted Schedule 20 herb under the UK Medicines Act, meaning it can only be used by qualified practitioners, and at a limited dose internally.

Externally it has a great reputation for combating warts. The bright orange sap, almost fluorescent it is so bright, is best used fresh dabbed onto warts daily. Avoid getting it elsewhere as when it dries it stains the skin a dark brown colour. The plant is very easy to grow and will self-seed readily. The yellow flowers are quite pretty and enjoyed by bees.

My favourite way to preserve and use this plant is to tincture it from freshly harvested leaves each year. Then it can be included in a cream or gel.

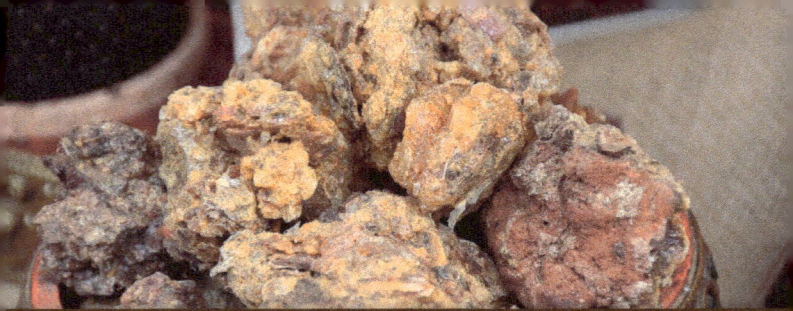

Myrrh sap resin
Commiphora myrrha

This is the resin from the sap of the Commiphora tree which grows in hot countries such as Africa. Sold as hard resinous chunks of dried sap, high strength alcohol (90%) is needed to dissolve it to liquid form. Alternatively it is available as a thick essential oil.

Research shows activity against staphylococcus aureus comparable to antibiotics[28].

In vitro testing supports histamine blocking effects, therefore allergic skin reactions can be reduced symptomatically by topical use[29]. This makes it useful in cases of allergic eczema which has become infected for instance.

One of the best anti-fungal, anti-microbial herbs to include in a cream especially when combined with other herbs such as thyme, garlic or oregano, working in synergy, studies confirm the effects against many pathogens[30].

28 Alotaibi, G., 'An in-vitro study to test antimicrobial effects of commiphora myrrha in comparison to biocides', n.d.,
29 Shin, J Y, et. al., 'Commiphora Myrrha Inhibits Itch-associated Histamine and IL-31 Production in Stimulated Mast Cells'. *Experimental and Therapeutic Medicine* 18, no. 3: 1914–20
30 ResearchGate. '(PDF) Antifungal Activity of Commiphora Myrrha L. against Some Air Fungi'. Accessed 7 September 2020.

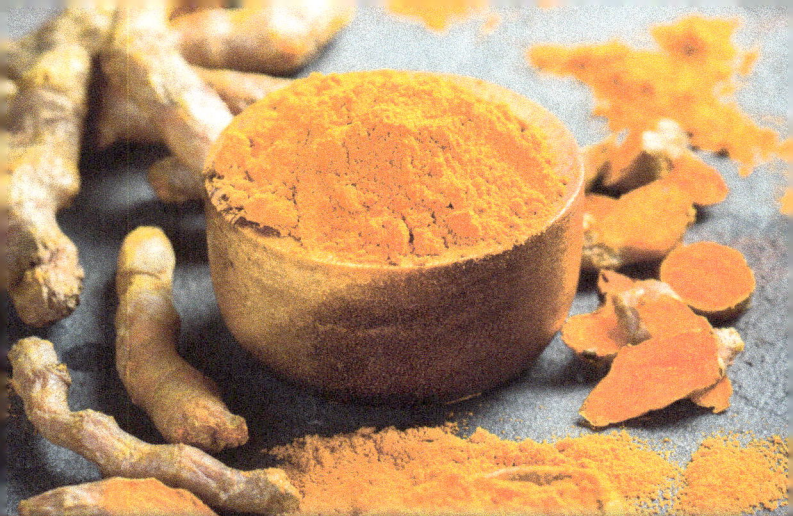

Turmeric
Curcuma longa

Turmeric will stain the skin, there is no doubt about this. Whether used as powder added to a cream, essential oil, or tincture. However, the benefits of this rhizome are far reaching, both internally and externally. I have found staining is minimised by cleaning the skin with cider vinegar each morning, following application of a turmeric cream overnight, though care does need to be taken if using on the face, plus use old bedding you don't mind being ruined! Studies show turmeric having anti-inflammatory, anti-microbial, anti-cancer, anti-acne effects, and improvement of solar keratosis spots[31].

31 Zaman, S, and Akhtar N., 'Effect of Turmeric (Curcuma Longa Zingiberaceae) Extract Cream on Human Skin Sebum Secretion'. *Trop. J. Pharm.* Res. 12, no. 5: 665–69

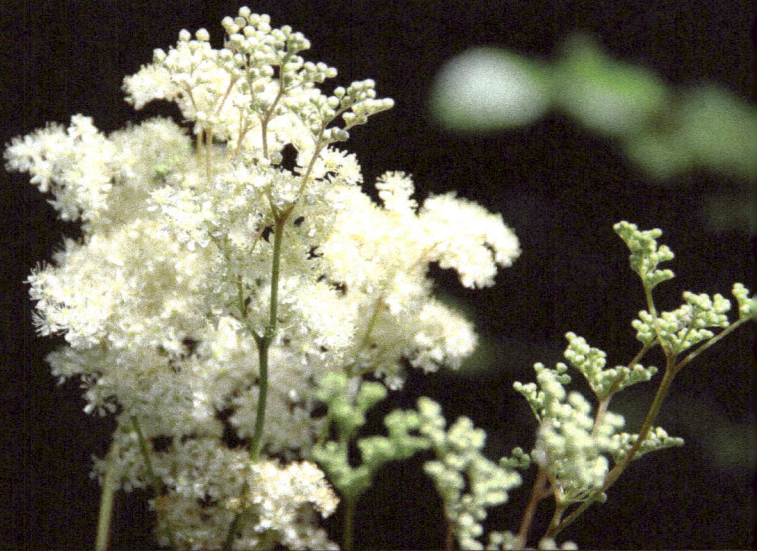

Meadowsweet
Filipendula ulmaria

Meadowsweet with its frothy cream flowers and the scent of almonds is a common sight in summer along country lanes, and it especially likes to grow along river banks. The flowers and leaves contain salicin which is the natural pain relieving molecule used and copied to make acetyl-salicylic acid, the synthetic version, aspirin. Unlike the synthetic version, meadowsweet does not irritate the stomach; in fact it has the opposite effect in that it is known for its antacid anti-inflammatory action. Used in a cream, usually as tincture or tea in the water portion, it has some pain relieving benefits that can be helpful for sore muscles, bruising and general aches and pains.

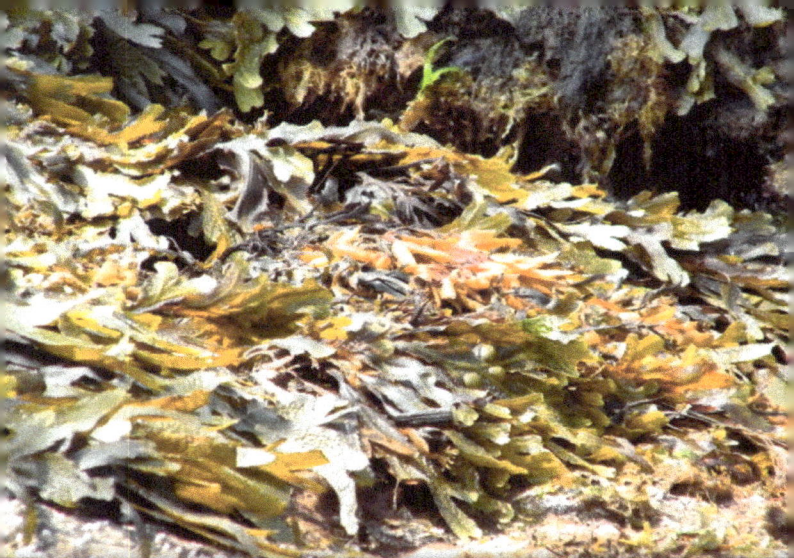

Bladderwrack seaweed
Fucus vesiculosis

The polysaccharides in seaweeds promote skin repair and maintenance, a short study on *Fucus*, bladderwrack seaweed extract at 1% in a gel showed considerable improvement in skin thickness after 5 weeks[32].

In my experience, seaweed extracts are highly susceptible to spoilage due to their water attracting polysaccharides. I have found tinctures to be far the easiest way to add their benefits to a cream. Alternatively, for a quick and easy option, you can purchase seaweed and aloe gel ready-made, to which you can add your own extra tinctures or essential oils.

32 Fujimura, T. et.al.,'Treatment of Human Skin with an Extract of Fucus Vesiculosus Changes Its Thickness and Mechanical Properties'. *Journal of Cosmetic Science* 53, no. 1: 1–9.

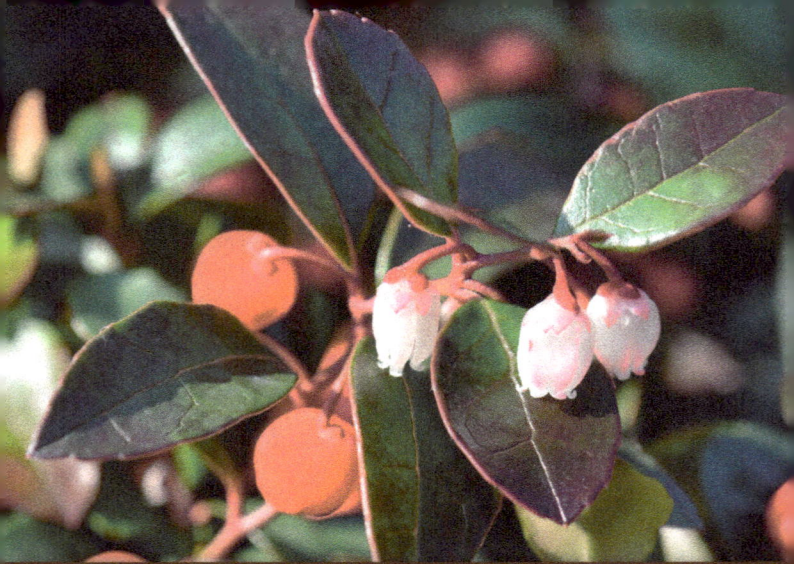

Wintergreen
Gaultheria procumbens

Wintergreen oil has a long traditional use for pain relief when applied topically. This low growing shrub produces beautiful red berries enhancing any garden, the leaves and twigs are used either to make essential oil, with that familiar antiseptic smell, a tincture, or a macerated oil. Water extractions are not usually as effective. The plant is high in salicylates and procyanidins which are believed to be part of the anti-inflammatory and analgesic action[33,34].

33 Michel, P. et.al.,'Polyphenolic Profile, Antioxidant and Anti-Inflammatory Activity of Eastern Teaberry (Gaultheria Procumbens L.) Leaf Extracts'. *Molecules* 19, no. 12
34 Michel, P, et.al., 'Salicylate and Procyanidin-Rich Stem Extracts of Gaultheria Procumbens L. Inhibit Pro-Inflammatory Enzymes and Suppress Pro-Inflammatory and Pro-Oxidant Functions of Human Neutrophils Ex Vivo'. *International Journal of Molecular Sciences* 20, no. 7

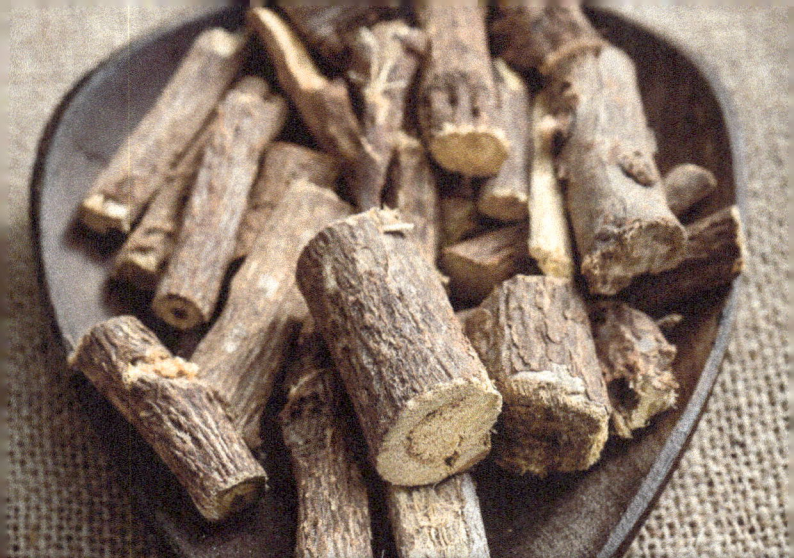

Liquorice
Glycyrrhiza glabra

Usually the root of this plant is used, although the leaves can be used and contain good amounts of anti-inflammatory polyphenols[35] well known for use in food, particularly confectionery, the flavour is very sweet and can be used to make medicines more palatable.

Used on the skin the main influence is anti-inflammatory[36].

Studies also show constituents in liquorice help with hyperpigmentation disorders such as melasma[37].

35 Siracusa, L, et.al., 'Phytocomplexes from Liquorice (Glycyrrhiza Glabra L.) Leaves...'. *Fitoterapia* 82, no. 4: 546–56.
36 Saeedi, M. et.al., 'The Treatment of Atopic Dermatitis with Licorice Gel'. *The Journal of Dermatological Treatment* 14, no. 3:153–57
37 ResearchGate. '(PDF) *Glabrene and Isoliquiritigenin as Tyrosinase Inhibitors from Licorice Roots*'.

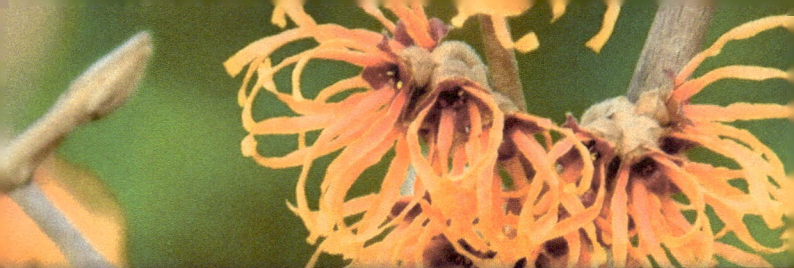

Witch hazel
Hammamelis virginiana

Witch hazel is available as a tincture, but usually commonly used as a hydrosol. A traditional remedy bought in small bottles in chemists for many years to use dabbed on bruises, the astringent properties tone and tighten tissues making it a valuable addition to creams for varicose veins[38].

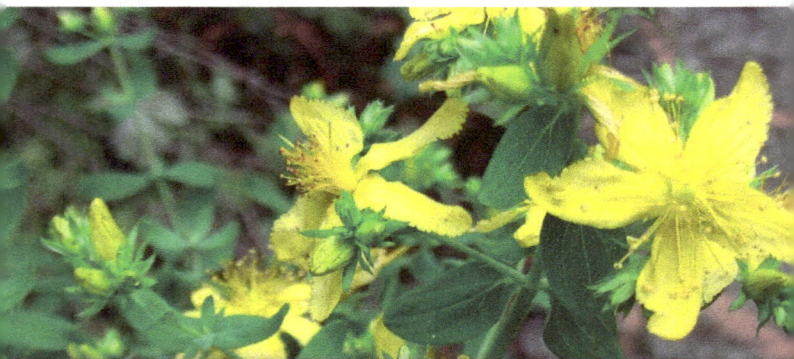

St. John's Wort
Hypericum perforatum

The fresh flowers and buds are generally used, along with a few top leaves and traditionally macerated in an oil to extract the constituents. The oil will turn a deep red as the extracts are drawn out. St John's wort oil is used to speed up healing of scrapes and grazes[39] and as a nerve pain reliever. It makes a very good addition to a pain relieving cream as the oil portion. It is also known to be of benefit against the cold sore virus[40], so can be included in a lip balm, often alongside lemon balm essential oil which is also shown to be anti-viral.

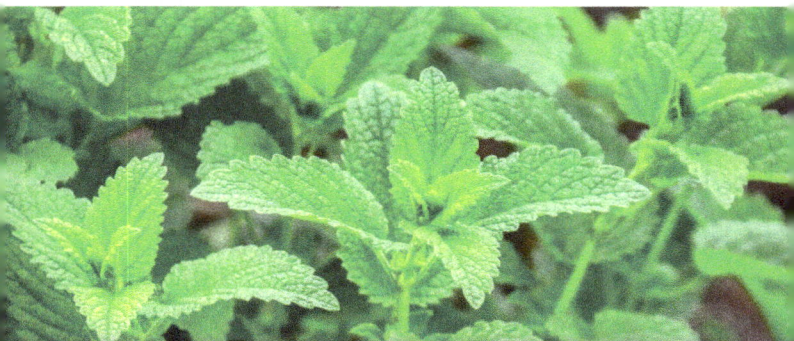

Lemon balm
Melissa officinalis

Hydrosol, tincture, and essential oil are all beneficial in particular against the cold sore virus[41]. A general antiseptic and anti-inflammatory benefit is also gained. Extracts of Lemon balm have been shown to improve skin elasticity when taken internally, and to give some UV protection when used externally.

38 Mackay, D. 'Hemorrhoids and Varicose Veins: A Review of Treatment Options'. *Alt. Med. Rev.* 6: 126–40.
39 Çobanoğlu, A, and Merdiye Ş., 'The Effect of Hypericum Perforatum Oil on the Healing Process in the Care of Episiotomy Wounds...' *Eur. J. Int. Med.* 34: 995.
40 Clewell, A, et.al., 'Efficacy and Tolerability Assessment of a Topical Formulation Containing Copper Sulfate and Hypericum Perforatum on Patients with Herpes Skin Lesions...'. *J.D.D.* 11: 209–15.
41 Mazzanti, G. et.al., 'Inhibitory Activity of Melissa Officinalis L. Extract on Herpes Simplex Virus Type 2 Replication'. *Nat. Prod. Res.* 22, no. 16: 1433–40.

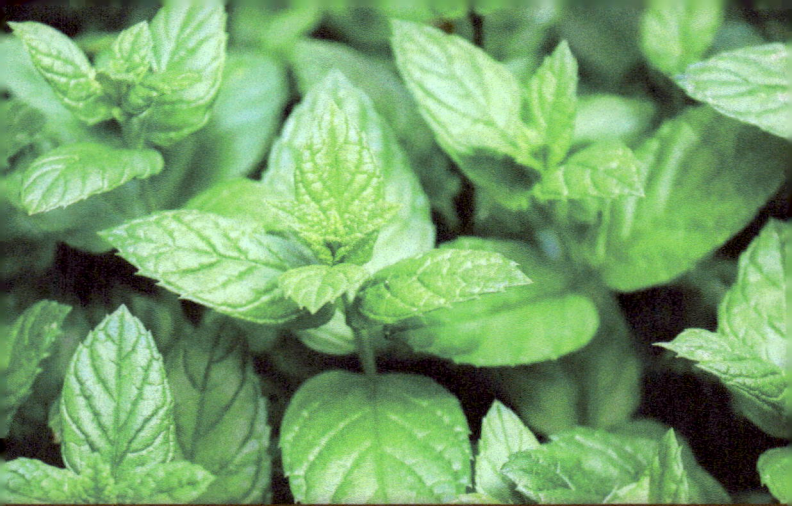

Peppermint
Mentha piperita

Traditional use for most types of mint is digestive and as a tea to ease trapped wind, which it does very well. Less known is the topical use as an anti-itch herb. Whatever the reason for the itchy skin, mint cools and soothes, giving symptomatic relief whilst the root cause is treated. Any kind of mint will work, though peppermint is the strongest[42].

It is worth noting that salves and oil based preparations may worsen itching due to their warming effects by occlusion or temporary pore blocking. Gels are cooling, with creams being closer to neutral the next choice. You can also use mint in a bath, often useful with oats, or make a herb tea as a wash.

42 Elsaie, L. T, et.al., 'Effectiveness of Topical Peppermint Oil on Symptomatic Treatment of Chronic Pruritus'. *Clin.Cos. & Inv. Derm* 9: 333–38.

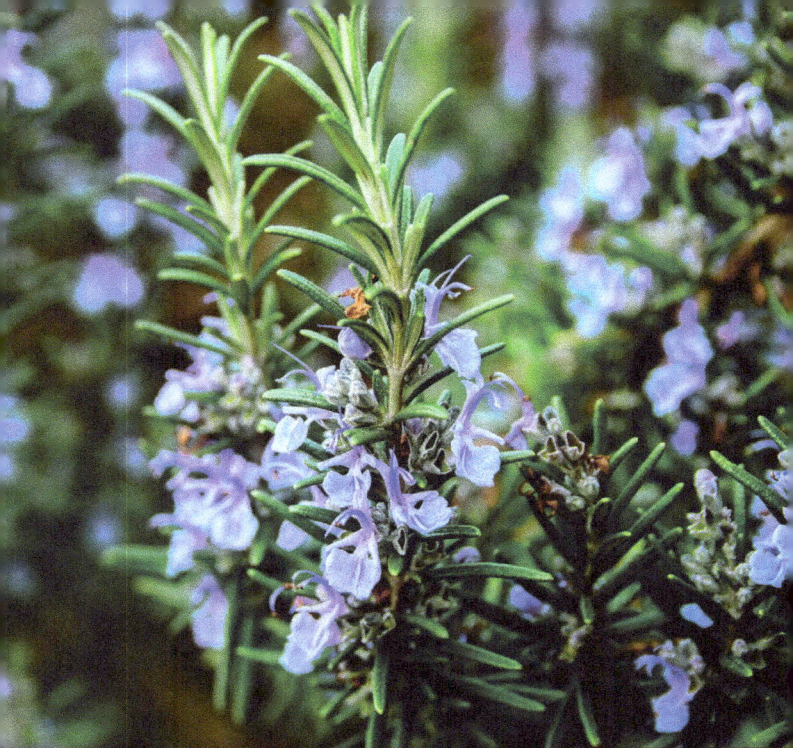

Rosemary
Rosmarinus officinalis (Salvia rosmarinus)

Rosemary macerated oil or diluted Rosemary essential oil has been shown to help with pain relief when applied to the skin[43]. The oil applied to the scalp in male pattern baldness showed some improvement when used over several months[44].

43 Keshavarzian, S, and Nahid S. 'Comparison of the Effect of Topical Application of Rosemary and Menthol for Musculoskeletal Pain in Hemodialysis Patients'. *Iran.J.Nurs.& Midwif Res.* 22:: 436
44 Panahi, Y. et.al., 'Rosemary Oil vs Minoxidil 2% for the Treatment of Androgenetic Alopecia: A Randomized Comparative Trial'. *Skinmed* 13, no. 1: 15–21.

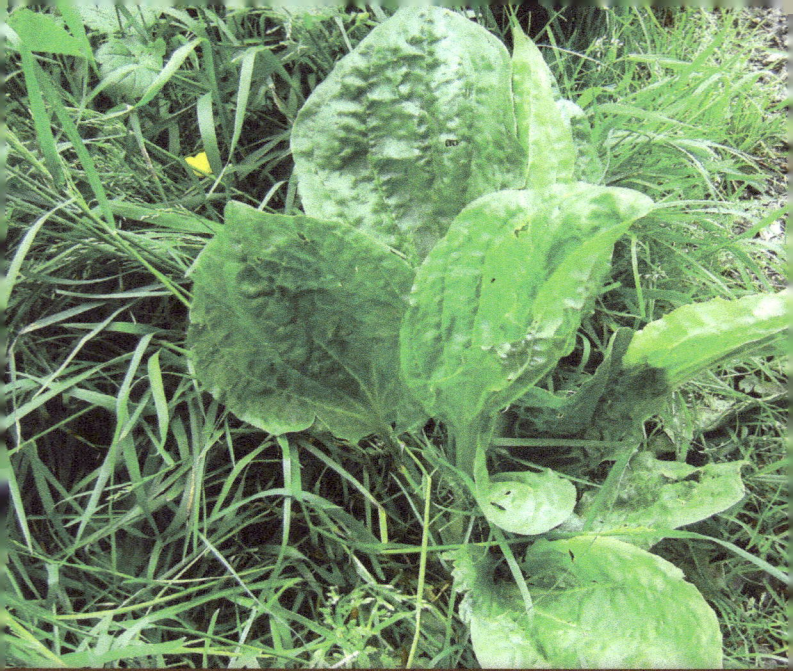

Plantain
Plantago spp.

A soothing, demulcent herb. The leaves of all types are often used as a great first aid remedy for insect stings, bites and nettle stings. Far more effective than using a dock leaf. Crush or chew a leaf and place on the area to immediately reduce pain and inflammation. Internally this herb is often used for calming irritation in the throat, especially dry coughs, and for acid reflux. There is also some antimicrobial effect[45]. Use in creams as the tincture portion, or water/hydrosol portion.

45 Adom. S. et.al., 'Chemical constituents and medical benefits of Plantago major' *J. Biomed & Pharmacother.* 96: 348-360.

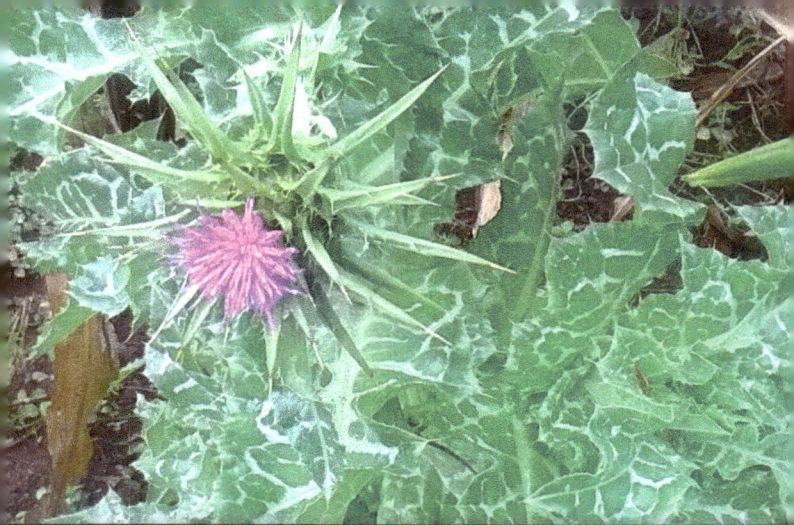

Milk thistle
Silybum marianum/Carduus marianus

The seeds of this beautiful though fiercely prickly member of the thistle family are most commonly known as a liver support remedy.

However, a clinical trial of patients with vitiligo found that there was a significant improvement when this herb was taken orally alongside UV treatment[46].

In vitro studies have also shown a measure of UV protection on human skin cells, including solar keratosis and the ageing acceleration associated with sun exposure when used on the skin[47].

46 Jowkar, F. et.al.,'Can We Consider Silymarin as a Treatment Option for Vitiligo? ...'. *J. Derm. Treat.* 31, no. 3: 256–60.
47 Vostálová, J. et.al., 'Skin Protective Activity of Silymarin and Its Flavonolignans'. *Molecules* 24, no. 6

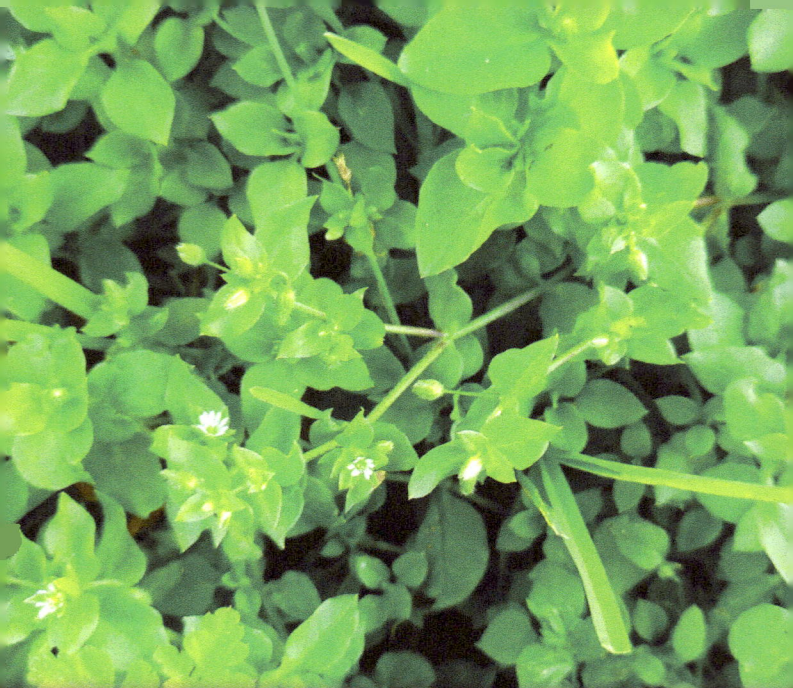

Chickweed
Stellaria media

This small plant which grows low to the ground is a treasure of the herbal medicine dispensary. The aerial parts (all above ground parts) can be used as freshly squeezed juice which can be done by crushing and squeezing by hand, tincture or macerated oil. The traditional use for anti-inflammatory, reducing itching and cooling effects is suitable in creams, water extract washes (teas) or gels.

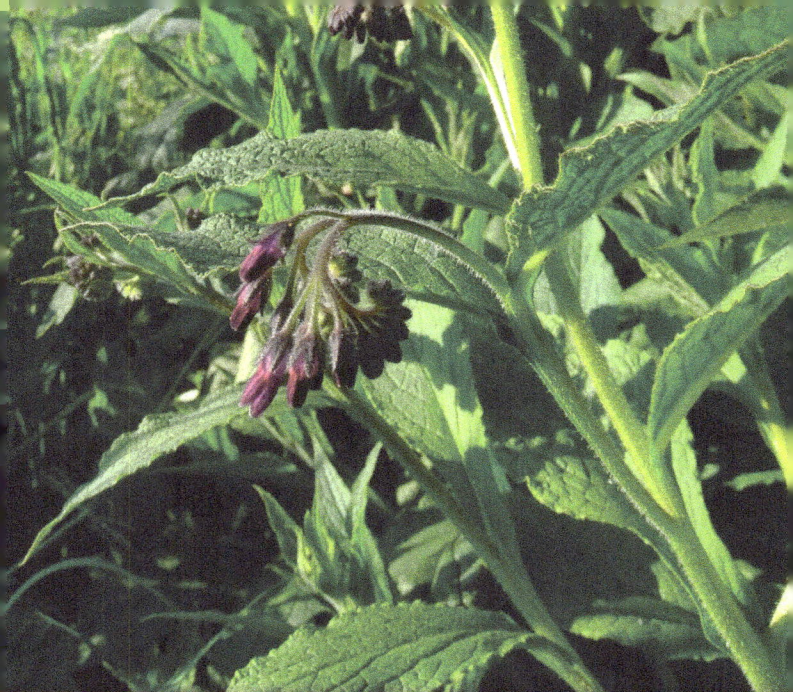

Comfrey
Symphytum officinalis

The old country name of *knitbone* gives a clue as to the value of the Comfrey plant in healing from the skin, to deeper tissues, and traditionally even bones. These days if you had a bone break unsuitable for having a plaster fitted, such as a toe, it certainly wouldn't harm you to use comfrey in some form to help healing. Studies support the benefits of comfrey to speed up healing of tissues[48].

48 Koll, R., et.al., 'Efficacy and Tolerance of a Comfrey Root Extract ... in the Treatment of Ankle Distorsions: ...'. *Phytomedicine* 11, no. 6: 470–77.

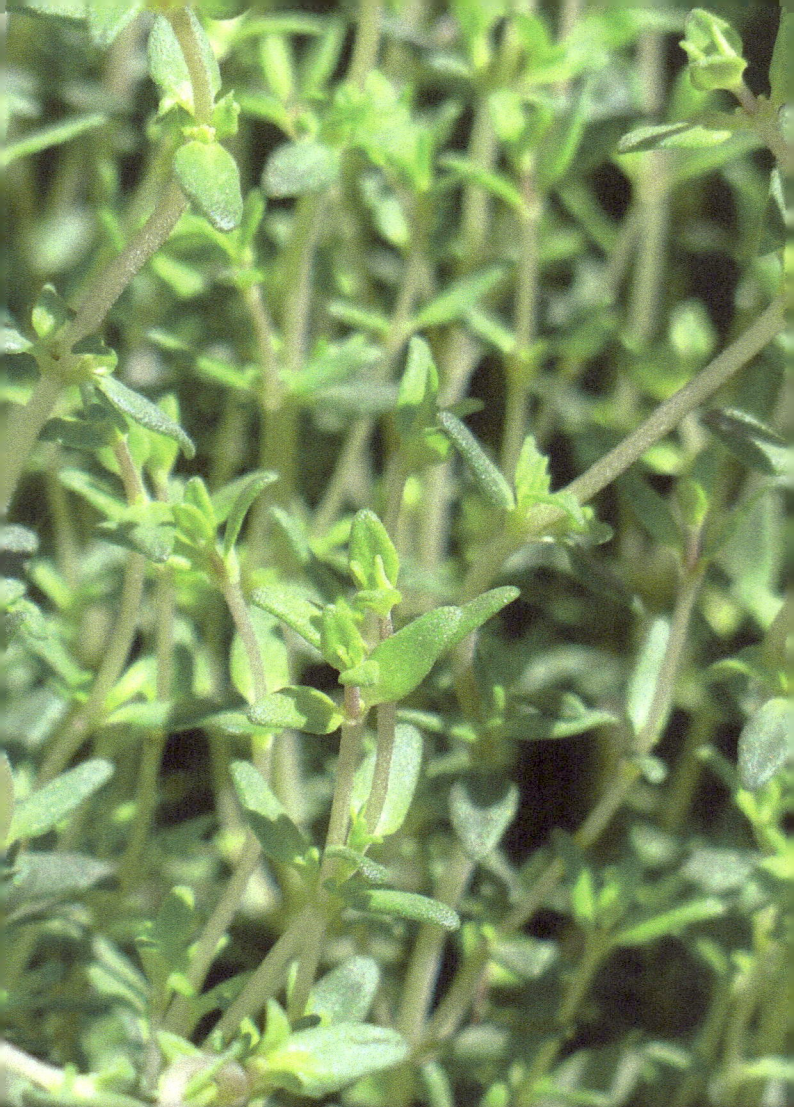

Thyme
Thymus vulgaris

There are many varieties of Thyme, with the common use as an internal or external anti-microbial herb in cases of sore throat, respiratory infections, skin infections or digestive infections. Of particular interest is the function of inhibition of the efflux pump by thyme. The efflux pump is a reaction I visualise to be a bit like a human vomit reflex, when you have a tummy bug your body vomits out the pathogen to recover. Some bacteria 'vomit' out substances which are a danger to them such as antibiotics, which is one reason why antibiotic resistance is more prevalent, bacteria learn. Thyme has been shown to switch off this efflux pump ability in some bacteria, therefore opening it to being eradicated by thyme itself, and other antibacterial agents. Therefore tenacious infections which resist orthodox antibiotics could also benefit from use in synergy[49].

Externally it has shown protective effects against UV light[50].

In vitro studies on a variety of skin pathogens, both bacterial and fungal, such as Staphylococcus aureus and ringworm, show excellent results in prevention and clearance, with the water soluble fraction and essential oil being the most effective. Therefore tinctures, hyrdosols, essential oils and teas, blended into a cream for skin absorption and adherence will produce good results[51].

49 Salehzadeh, A. et.al., 'The Effect of Thyme (Thymus Vulgaris) Extract on the Expression of NorA Efflux Pump Gene in Clinical Strains of Staphylococcus Aureus', *J. Genet. Resour.*, 1 January 2018, 26–36.
50 Cornaghi, L. et.al., 'Effects of UV Rays and Thymol/Thymus Vulgaris L. ...'. *Cells Tissues Organs* 201, no. 3: 180–92.
51 ResearchGate. '(PDF) *Antimicrobial Activity of Topical Formulations Containing Thymus Vulgaris Essential Oil on Major Pathogens Causing Skin Diseases*'

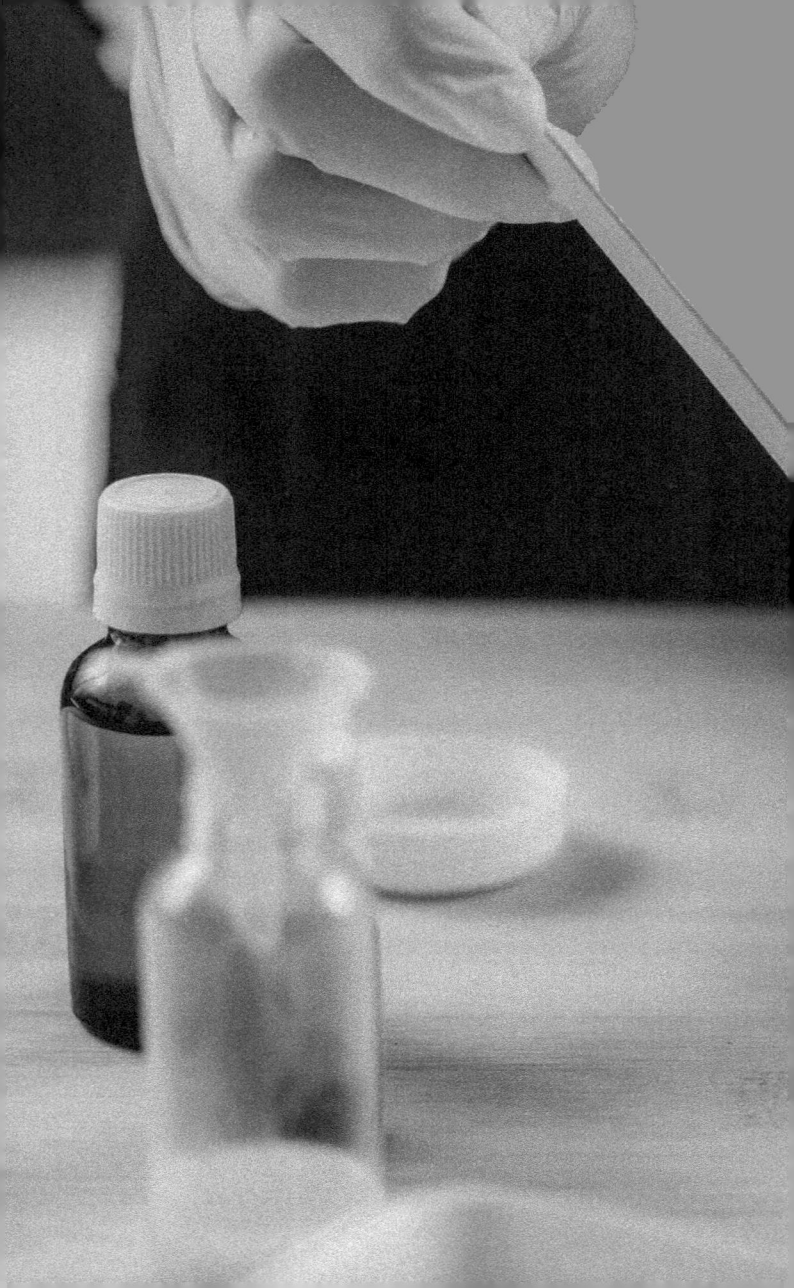

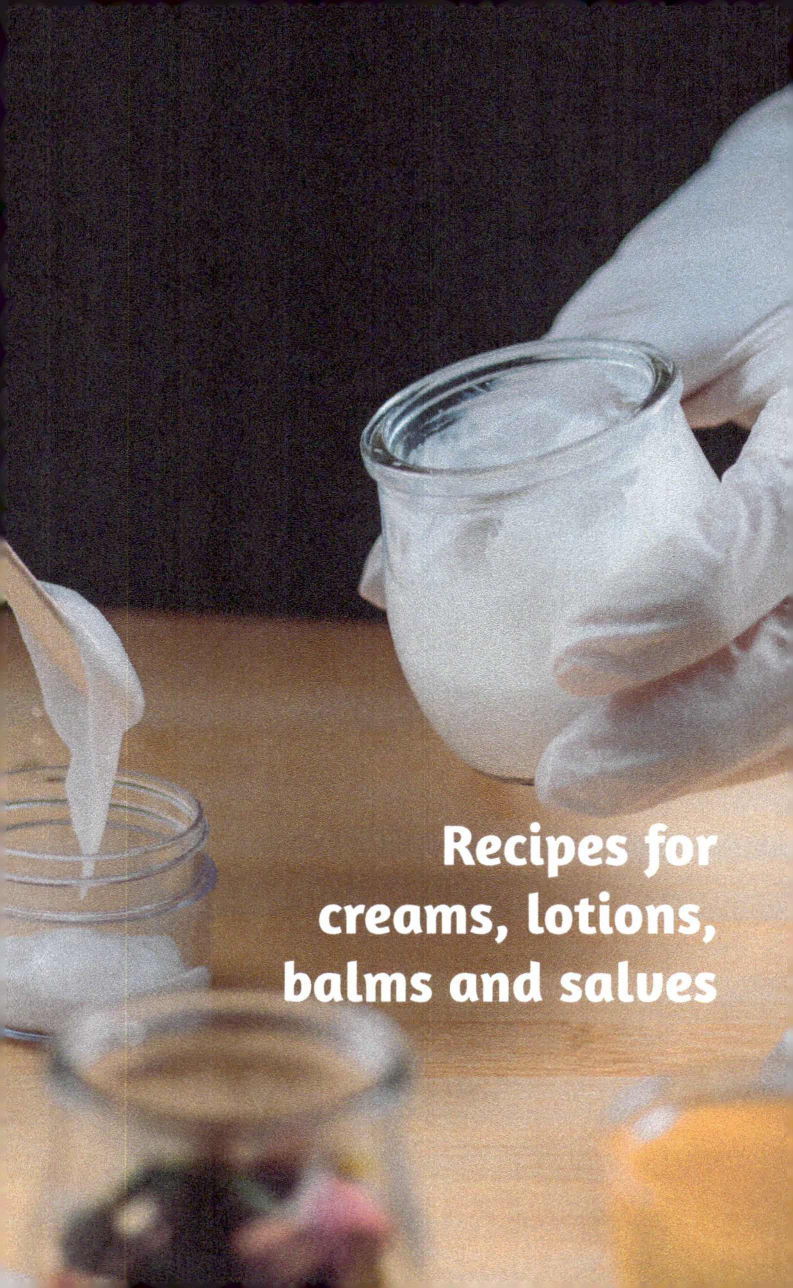

Recipes for creams, lotions, balms and salves

A few basic recipes you can adapt with different herbs for different uses. Some tips for the below recipes:

- All formulas make 50ml volume.
- All measurements are in grams unless drops of essential oil or CO_2.
- As these are natural extracts, room temperature can influence the product, making it softer or harder. You may also find the creams continue to set and thicken slightly during the first 24 hours after making.
- Sterilise jars, equipment and utensils to help combat spoilage, either by wiping with alcohol, or immersing in very hot water.
- Close lids on jars or bottles only after cooled to avoid condensation building on the inside of lids and increasing the chances of mould, unless using airless pumps.
- You don't need to buy in all the ingredients for these recipes. Choose one or two recipes and adapt to thicken or thin each time, or keep as a base cream to add extra ingredients as needed.

A note on alcohol tinctures

If you prefer to avoid the use of alcohol extracts in these recipes it can easily be done by substituting the same amount for extra hydrosol, tea or plant juice. You will need to increase the preservative by doubling it or keep the cream in the fridge. Alternatively glycerite could be substituted in which case the preservative won't need increasing. Add that to the water stage. The latter may alter the consistency a little.

Image on the right. From top to bottom: salve, whipped butter, thick cream, light cream, lotion and mousse lotion

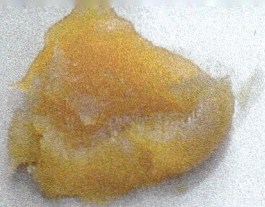

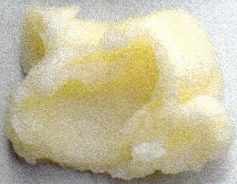

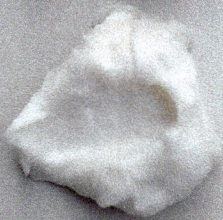

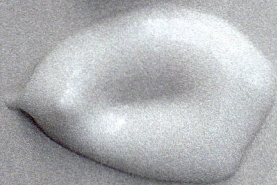

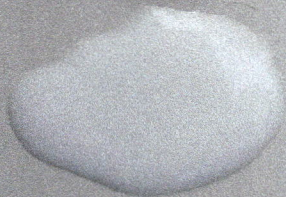

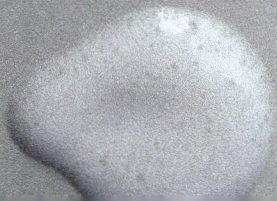

Gentle salve ointment

Non-sting.
Great for small
children, and big.

Ingredients

- 35 g Oil or combination of oils
- 10 g Lecithin emulsifier (syrup consistency, or macerate granules in oil overnight)
- 10 g Candelilla wax

Optional extras

- 3 drops of CO_2 extract
- Essential oil, or combination of oils 3 - 6 drops

Method

Gently melt stage one oils and waxes in a pan until fully liquid (approx. 70°C). Remove from heat, stir well until 55°C or until they just begin to show signs of thickening, then add stage two ingredients if using. Stir in well and pour into jars to set. Allow to cool before putting lids on to avoid condensation forming on the inside of caps, as this would promote bacterial or fungal growth. The finished product is a dark amber colour.

This recipe is a favourite with many people I know, and has been particularly effective at healing and prevention of small but painful splits in the skin due to constant cold or wetting, such as finger splits or vaginal or anal tissue inflammation from continence issues.

Whipped balm butter

No emulsifier necessary

Ingredients

- 20 g Shea butter or coconut oil
- 30 g Oil or combination of oils
- 1 g Candelilla wax

Optional extras

- 3 - 5 drops of essential oil or combination of oils
- 3 drops of CO_2 extract

Method

Weigh ingredients into a pan and melt until a temperature of 70°C is reached to ensure all fatty acids are dissolved. Remove from the heat and whisk until opaque.

Place in the fridge or a cold place for half an hour. Remove and whisk again. Place in the fridge again, whisk and repeat this process until a thick buttery consistency is reached. Pot in a glass jar.

This is a nice soft nourishing buttery balm for things such as nappy balm when calendula oil is used (no essential oils), or a gardeners hand balm with comfrey oil and rosemary or lavender essential oil, or a chest balm for respiratory conditions with eucalyptus essential oil.

Thick cream

Ingredients

Water solubles
- 40 g Hydrosol of choice
- 5 g Tincture
- 5 g Glycerine or glycerite (previously macerated with herbs)
- 1 g Preservative if using (such as Geogard) or
  20 drops if using liquid such as Eco-preservative

Fat solubles
- 10 g Oil or combination of oils
- 10 g Cocoa butter
- 5 g Vegetal emulsifier

Optional extras

- 3 - 5 drops of essential oil or blend of essential oils
- 3 drops of CO_2 extract
- Half a teaspoon of colloidal oatmeal powder blended with one teaspoon of glycerine added to the water portion before blending with the oil portion. Turmeric powder, half a teaspoon blended in final cream.

Method

Place the water soluble ingredients in one pan, and the fat solubles in another (except essential oils and CO2 extracts), or a heat proof bowl over a pan of hot water, or a bain marie double boiler to avoid over heating ingredients.

Melt and heat both pans to the same temperature to ensure all fatty acids are liquid: this needs to be approximately 70°C for both. The water solubles should not be cooler than the fats when you blend together or you may run the risk of some fat components solidifying quickly before there is chance to blend, resulting in a grainy or gritty product.

Stir together until the consistency starts to thicken.

Vegetal blends better if you whisk quickly for a minute initially, then stir slowly after that.

Check the temperature, and when it is down below 55°C add essential oils and stir in well. Pot up the creams. Store in a cool place out of the sun, you do not need to refrigerate.

This works well with anything that needs a good rich cream, or a base cream you can store and add 25% additional tinctures or oils at a later date. (not applicable if you have thinned the recipe down to start with)

Useful for psoriasis or eczema cream using mint hydrosol to combat itching, or anti-inflammatory rose water hydrosol, or colloidal oatmeal, as a soothing anti-inflammatory, oat CO_2 extract and chamomile essential oil.

You can make this cream thinner and lighter by doubling the amount of hydrosol in the same recipe, plus adding an extra 5g of tincture.

Light cream

Ingredients

You can make this cream thicker by increasing cocoa butter by 2 g

Water solubles
- 40 g Hydrosol of choice
- 3 g Tincture
- 1 g Preservative such as Geogard or 10 drops Preservative Eco

Fat solubles
- 2 g Cocoa butter
- 4 g Glyceryl citrate
- 4 g Cetyl alcohol
- 8 g Oil or combination of oils

Optional extras

- 3 - 5 drops of essential oil or blend of essential oils
- 3 drops of CO_2 extract
- Powders such as turmeric or colloidal oatmeal. Half a teaspoon. Easier blended with a little glycerine first to avoid lumps, added to final cream before potting up.

Method

Place the water soluble ingredients in one pan, and the fat solubles in another (except essential oils and CO_2 extracts), or a heat proof bowl over a pan of hot water, or a bain marie double boiler to avoid over heating ingredients.

Melt and heat both pans to the same temperature to ensure all fatty acids are liquid, this needs to be approximately 70°C for both. The water solubles should not be cooler than the fats when you blend together or you may run the risk of some fat components solidifying quickly before there is chance to blend, resulting in a grainy or gritty product. Stir together until the consistency starts to thicken. Add optional extras when temperature drops below 55°C.

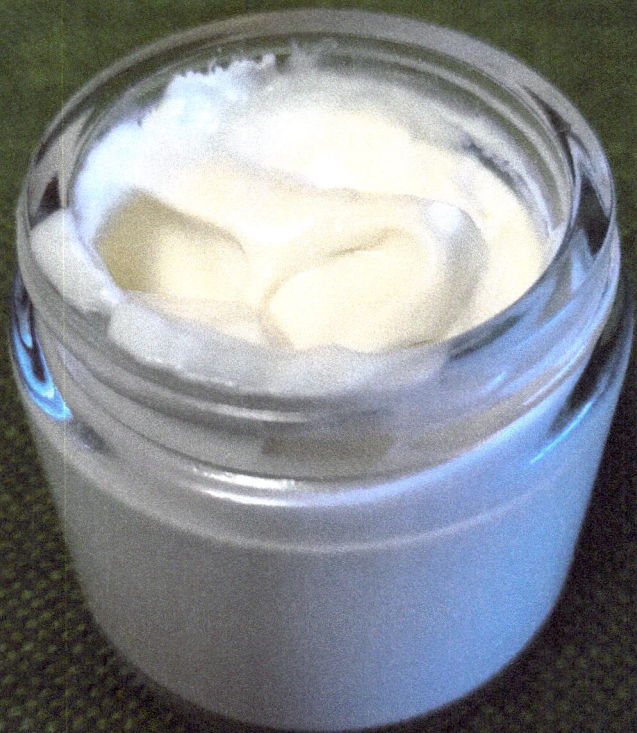

Lotion

Ingredients

Water solubles
- 33 g Hydrosol of choice
- 3 g Tincture
- 1 g Preservative such as Geogard or 20 drops of liquid preservative

Fat solubles
- 2 g Shea butter
- 5 g Glyceryl citrate
- 7 g Cetearyl alcohol
- 7 g Oil or blend of oils

Optional extras

- 3 - 5 drops of essential oil or blend of essential oils
- 3 drops of CO_2 extract

Method

Melt and heat both pans to the same temperature to ensure all fatty acids are liquid; this needs to be approximately 70°C for both. The water solubles should not be cooler than the fats when you blend together or you may run the risk of some fat components solidifying quickly before there is chance to blend, resulting in a grainy or gritty product.

Stir together until the consistency starts to thicken. Add optional extras when temperature drops below 55°C.

The lotion can be made thicker by increasing cetearyl alcohol emulsifier by 5g. The thicker version works well with anything that needs a good rich cream, or a base cream you can store and add 25% additional tinctures or oils at a later date (not applicable if you have thinned the recipe down to start with).

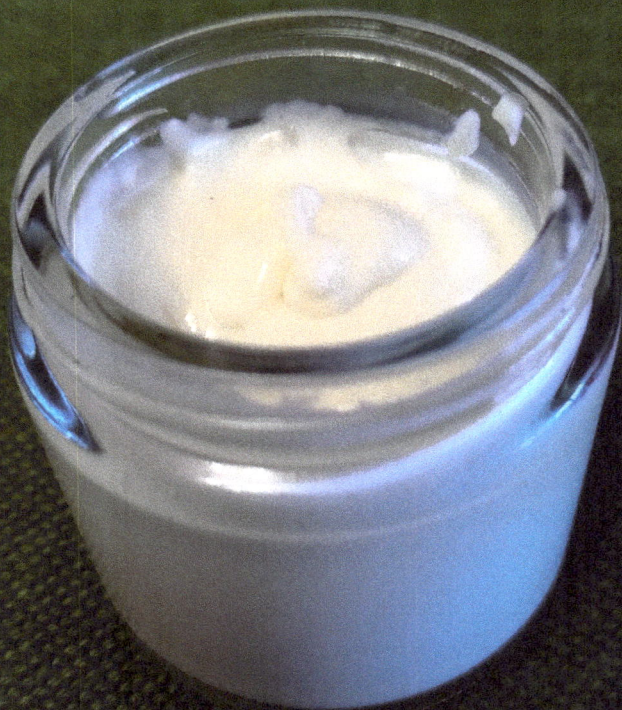

Mousse-type lotion

Ideal for light and gentle needs such as fragile skin

Ingredients

Water solubles
- 30 g Hydrosol of choice
- 3 g Tincture
- 10 drops of preservative or 0.5 g powdered

Fat solubles
- 3 g Shea butter
- 6 g Coco glucoside
- 5 g Cetyl alcohol
- 10 g Oil or combination of oils

Optional extras

- 3 - 5 drops of essential oil or blend of essential oils
- 3 drops of CO_2 extract

Method

Melt and heat both pans to the same temperature to ensure all fatty acids are liquid; this needs to be approximately 70°C for both. The water solubles should not be cooler than the fats when you blend together or you may run the risk of some fat components solidifying quickly before there is chance to blend, resulting in a grainy or gritty product.

Stir together until the consistency starts to thicken. Add optional extras when temperature drops below 55°C.

You will find this recipe foams up like a mousse.

Thin emulsion-type lotion

Uses natural lecithin

Ingredients

Water solubles
- 40 g Hydrosol of choice
- 7 g Tincture
- 10 drops of eco-preservative or 1 g Geogard preservative

Fat solubles
- 10 g Oil
- 7 g Cocoa butter
- 1 g Lecithin

Optional extras

- 3 - 5 drops of essential oil or blend of essential oils
- 3 drops of CO_2 extract

Method

Melt and heat both pans to the same temperature to ensure all fatty acids are liquid; this needs to be approximately 70°C for both. The water solubles should not be cooler than the fats when you blend together or you may run the risk of some fat components solidifying quickly before there is chance to blend, resulting in a grainy or gritty product.

Stir together until the consistency starts to thicken. Add optional extras when temperature drops below 55°C.

This emulsifier in a cream can seem quite gloopy when it first blends, stir till cool, then leave aside in a cool place for an hour, stir again and this will settle.

Aloe gel

Ingredients

- 50 g Aloe gel
- 5 g Tincture

Method

The easiest way to extract a good amount of gel from Aloe is to freeze the leaves in my experience (or quick cheat is to buy in ready-made gel to add your own extras). You can purchase Aloe and Seaweed gel ready-made, which has amazing healing and anti-inflammatory benefits.

A few drops of Lavender essential oil mixed in Aloe gel is the best minor burn relief I've tried.

A 10% addition of Myrrh tincture blended in Aloe gel makes a great anti-fungal foot gel. Include Peppermint essential oil and you have a refreshing anti-itch benefit too.

Image on the right. Top left clockwise: keratosis cream with calendula, chelidonium and turmeric essential oil: eczema cream with chamomile blue, and colloidal oats: psoriasis cream with liquorice, mint and chamomile: bruise cream with comfrey, daisy and witch hazel.

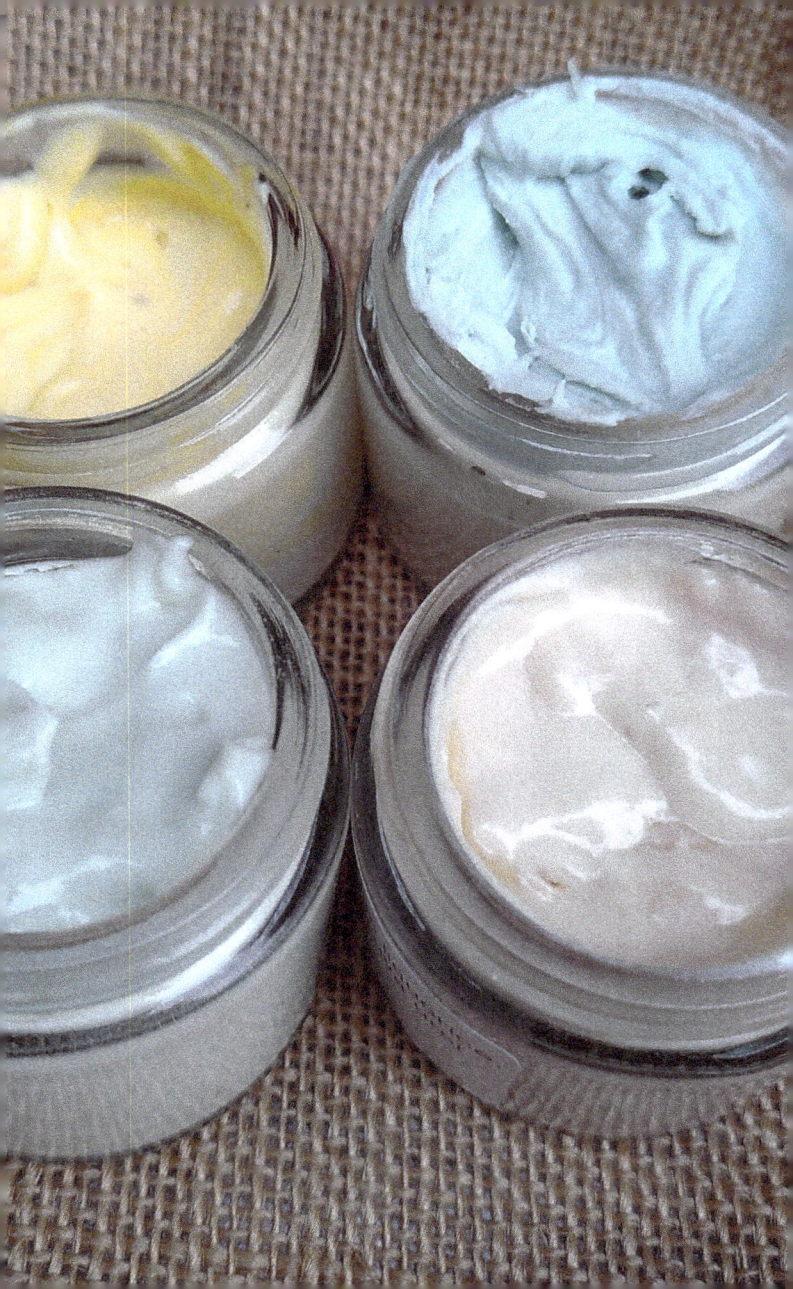

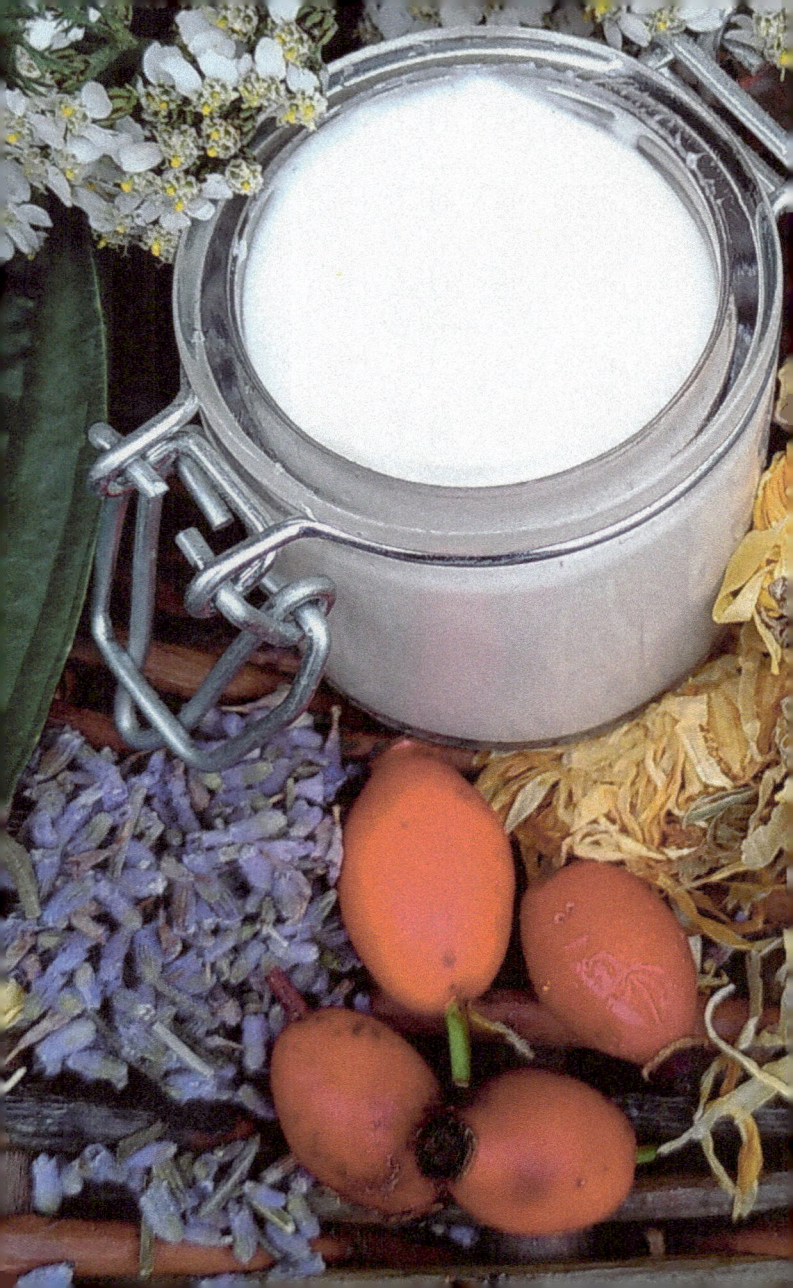

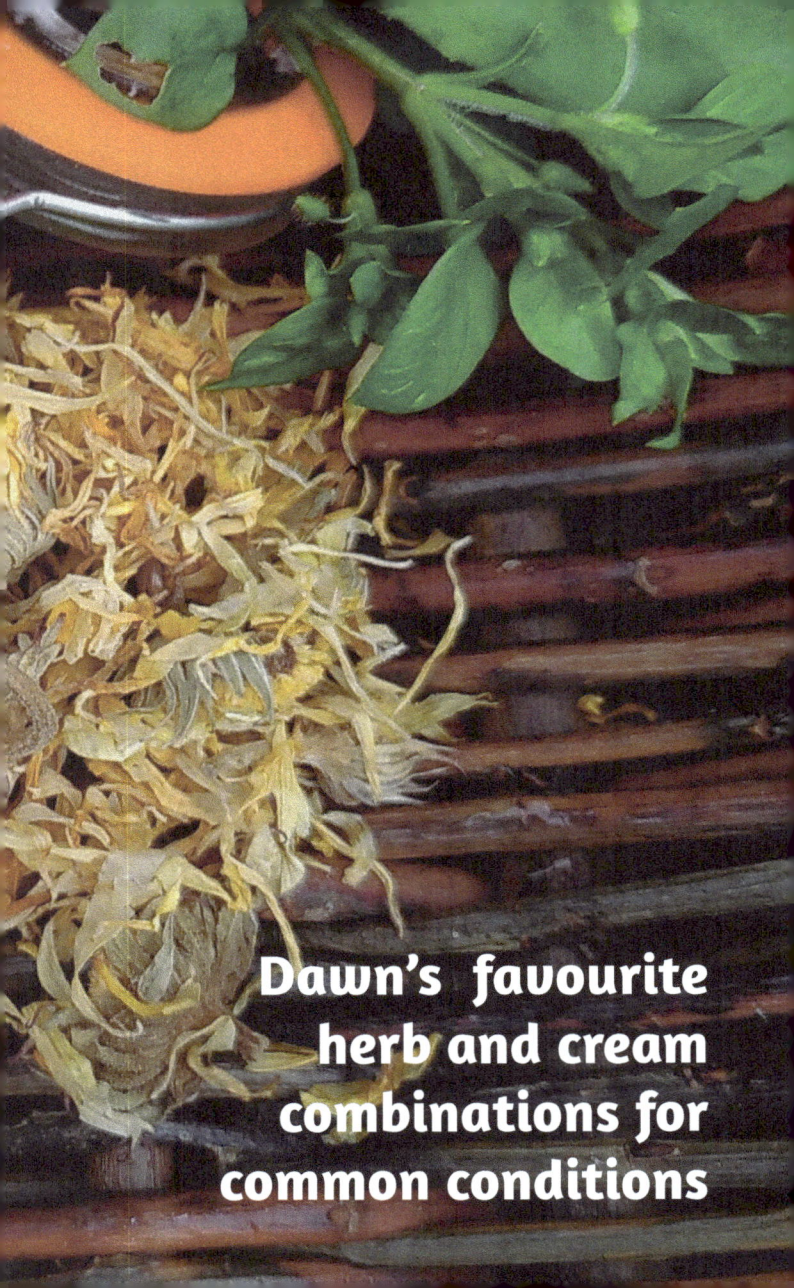

Dawn's favourite herb and cream combinations for common conditions

Antiseptic cream

with Rosemary hydrosol, Echinacea tincture, Lemon Balm oil and Thyme or Rosemary essential oil

Ingredients

Water solubles
- 40 g Rosemary hydrosol
- 3 g Echinacea tincture
- 10 drops of liquid Preservative Eco (Aromantic)

Oil solubles
- 2 g Cocoa butter
- 4 g Glyceryl citrate
- 4 g Cetyl alcohol (pellets)
- 8 g Lemon Balm macerated oil

Optional extras

After the cream is blended, add some optional extras: 2 drops of Thyme essential oil and 3 drops of Rosemary essential oil

Bruise cream

with Witch Hazel hydrosol, Daisy tincture, Comfrey and Calendula oil

Ingredients

Water solubles
- 40 g Witch Hazel hydrosol (distilled witch hazel)

- 3 g Daisy tincture (or arnica tincture)
- 10 drops of liquid Preservative Eco (Aromantic)

Oil solubles
- 2 g Cocoa butter
- 4 g Glyceryl citrate
- 4 g Cetyl alcohol (pellets)
- 5 g Comfrey macerated oil
- 5 g Calendula macerated oil

Optional extras

After the cream is blended, add some optional extras:
3 drops of Calendula CO^2 extract (optional)

Chest balm salve
for respiratory conditions with Rosemary oil, and
essential oils of Eucalyptus, Pine and Nutmeg

Ingredients

Oil solubles
- 35 g Macerated Rosemary oil
- 10 g Lecithin
- 10 g Candelilla wax

Optional extras

After melting and removing from heat, wait until temperature
drops to 50°C then add 5 drops each of essential oils of
Eucalyptus, Pine, Nutmeg, Rosemary, Juniper and Clove

Dermatitis anti-inflammatory cream
with Rose hydrosol, Chamomile tincture, Calendula oil

Ingredients

Water solubles
- 33 g Rosewater hydrosol
- 3 g Chamomile tincture
- 1 g Geogard ultra preservative

Oil solubles
- 2 g Shea butter
- 5g Glyceryl citrate
- 7g Cetearyl alcohol
- 7g Calendula macerated oil

Optional extras

After the cream is blended, add some optional extras: 3 drops each of Chamomile blue essential oil, and CO_2 Chamomile extract (optional)

Eczema cream or lotion
with peppermint hydrosol, chamomile tincture, oat CO2 or colloidal oat powder, and chamomile blue essential oil

Ingredients

Water solubles
- 40 g Peppermint hydrosol
- 3 g Chamomile tincture

- 5 g Chickweed pressed juice
- 3 g Plantago glycerite
- 2 g Geogard ultra preservative

Oil solubles
- 2 g Cocoa butter
- 4 g Glyceryl citrate
- 4 g Cetyl alcohol
- 8 g Comfrey macerated oil

Optional extras

After the cream is made, add some optional extras: 3 drops Oat CO^2 and/or half a teaspoon of colloidal oat powder mixed with a teaspoon of glycerine before blending.

Fungicidal cream
with tea tree or thyme hydrosol, myrrh or berberis tincture, thyme macerated oil and essential oil

Ingredients

Water solubles
- 40 g Tea tree hydrosol
- 5 g Berberis vulgaris tincture
- 5 g Thyme tincture
- 1 g Geogard ultra preservative

Oil solubles
- 10 g Cocoa butter
- 10 g Thyme macerated oil
- 5 g Vegetal emulsifier

Optional extras

After the cream is made, add some optional extras: 5 drops Thyme essential oil and/or 5 drops Myrrh essential oil

Gentle healing balm
for non-sting healing and protection of grazes (great for small kids, and big)

Ingredients

Oil solubles
- 20 g Cocoa butter
- 15 g Rosehip oil
- 15 g Comfrey macerated oil
- 1 g Candelilla wax

Optional extras

Optional extras added when temperature of melted oils drops to 50°C:

- 5 drops Helichrysum essential oil
- 5 drops Yarrow or Chamomile blue essential oil
- 3 drops of Calendula CO_2 extract

Please note that this recipe needs whisking.

Keratosis cream

with Rosemary (antioxidant) hydrosol, greater Celandine tincture, castor oil, Turmeric essential oil

Ingredients

Water solubles
- 40 g Rosemary hydrosol
- 3 g Chelidonium tincture (or Figwort/Scrophularia tincture if you can't get the former)
- 10 drops Preservative Eco

Oil solubles
- 2 g Cocoa butter
- 4 g Glyceryl Citrate
- 4 g Cetyl Alcohol
- 8 g Castor oil

Optional extras

Optional extras after blending cream:
- 5 drops Turmeric essential oil
- 3 drops Rosemary essential oil

Half a teaspoon of Turmeric powder first blended in a teaspoon of glycerine.

Please note that this will likely stain the skin and clothing.

Melasma cream

with rose hydrosol, berberis tincture, and chamomile and fennel essential oil

Ingredients

Water solubles
- 33 g Rosewater hydrosol
- 3 g Berberis tincture
- 20 drops Preservative Eco

Oil solubles
- 1 g Shea butter
- 5 g Glyceryl citrate
- 7 g Cetearyl alcohol
- 7 g Fennel seed macerated oil

Optional extras

Optional extras after blending cream:
- 3 drops Fennel essential oil
- 3 drops Chamomile blue essential oil

Pain relief cream

with aloe vera hydrosol, willow bark tincture, rosemary tincture, St. John's wort oil, and wintergreen essential oil

Ingredients

Water solubles
- 40 g Aloe vera hydrosol

- 5 g Willow bark tincture (or Atropa or Arnica or Aconite tincture if you can get this)
- 5 g Rosemary glycerite (previously made)
- 1 g Geogard Ultra

Oil solubles
- 10 g St John's wort oil (*Naturally Thinking* do expeller expressed seed oil, or use macerated oil)
- 10 g Cocoa butter
- 5 g Vegetal

Optional extras

Optional extras after blending cream:
- 10 drops Wintergreen essential oil
- 5 drops Nutmeg essential oil

Psoriasis cream

with Peppermint hydrosol, Berberis, or Liquorice and Reishi tincture, and Chamomile CO_2 extracts or essential oil

Ingredients

Water solubles
- 40 g Peppermint hydrosol
- 3 g Berberis tincture
- 3 g Reishi tincture
- 1 g Geogard Ultra preservative

Oil solubles
- 8 g Liquorice root macerated oil

- 4 g Glyceryl citrate
- 4 g Cetyl alcohol
- 2 g Cocoa butter

Optional extras

Optional extras after blending cream:
- 3 drops Chamomile blue essential oil
- 3 drops Peppermint essential oil (if skin is itchy)
- 3 drops Chamomile CO_2 extract

Salve for Split fingers & Gardeners hand protection

Ingredients

Oil solubles
- 35 g Comfrey macerated oil
- 10 g Lecithin emulsifier
- 10 g Candelilla wax

Optional extras

Optional extras added after melting and temperature of salve reduced to 50°C:
- 5 drops Calendula CO_2 extract
- 5 drops Lavender essential oil

Sunburn lotion

with Aloe and Lavender hydrosol, Milk thistle tincture, Rose glycerite and Lavender essential oil

Ingredients

Water solubles
- 35 g Aloe vera hydrosol
- 5 g Lavender tincture
- 3 g Milk thistle tincture
- 5 g Rose petal glycerite (previously made)
- 20 drops of Presevative Eco

Oil solubles
- 7 g Chamomile macerated oil
- 7 g Cetearyl alcohol
- 5 g Glyceryl citrate
- 2 g Cocoa butter

Optional extras

Optional extras after blending lotion:
- 5 drops of Lavender essential oil
- 2 drops Spearmint essential oil

Varicose vein lotion

with Witch hazel hydrosol, Horse chestnut tincture, St. John's wort oil

Ingredients

Water solubles
- 30 g Witch hazel hydrosol
- 3 g Horse chestnut tincture
- 10 drops Preservative Eco

Oil solubles
- 10 g St John's wort oil
- 6g Coco glucoside
- 5g Cetyl alcohol
- 3g Shea butter

Optional extras

Optional extras after blending lotion:
- 3 drops Peppermint essential oil (if skin is hot or itchy)
- 3 drops Calendula CO^2 extract

Wart remover cream

with Lemon balm hydrosol, greater Celandine or Thuja tincture, Myrrh essential oil

Ingredients

Water solubles
- 40 g Lemon balm hydrosol

- 5 g Thuja tincture
- 5 g Chelidonium tincture (or Lemon balm tincture)
- 1 g Geogard Ultra preservative

Oil solubles
- 10 g Rosemary macerated oil
- 10 g Shea butter
- 5 g Vegetal emulsifier

Optional extras

Optional extras after blending cream:

- 5 drops Myrrh essential oil
- 5 drops Rosemary essential oil

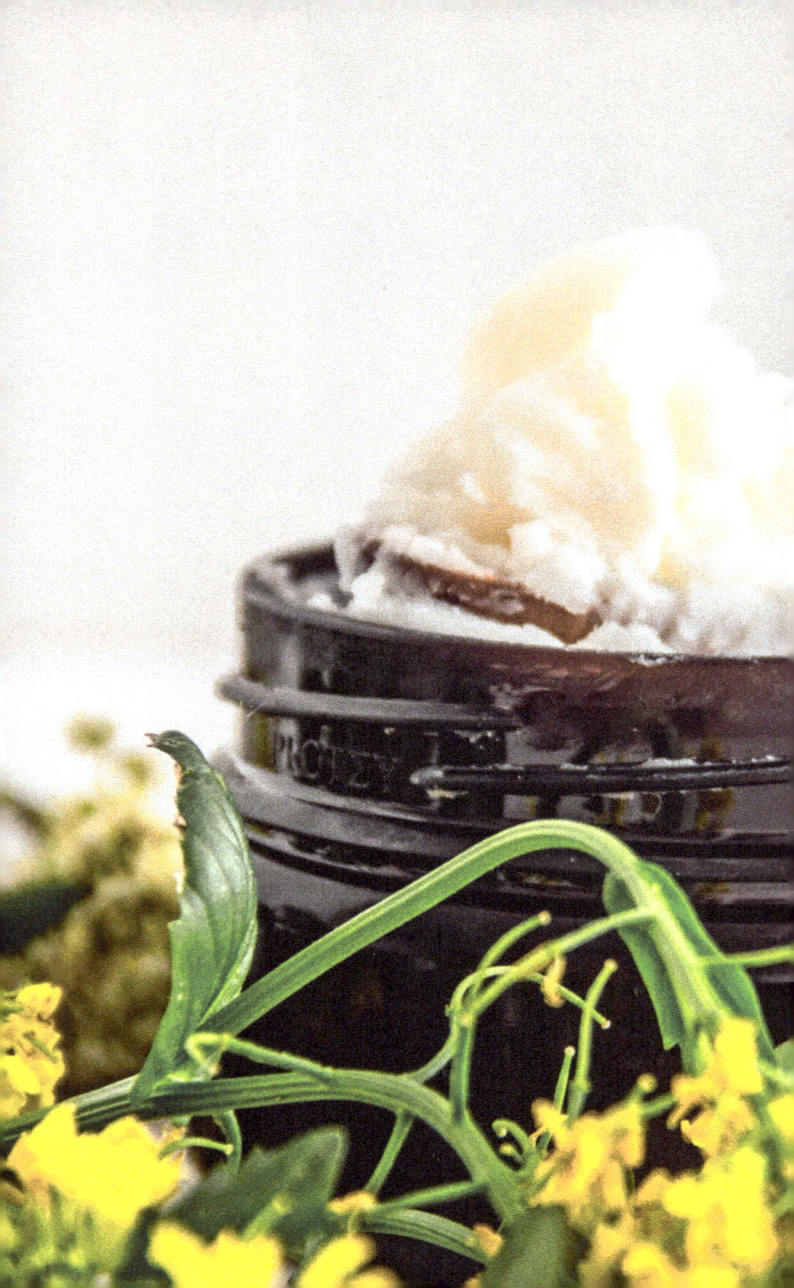

Troubleshooting

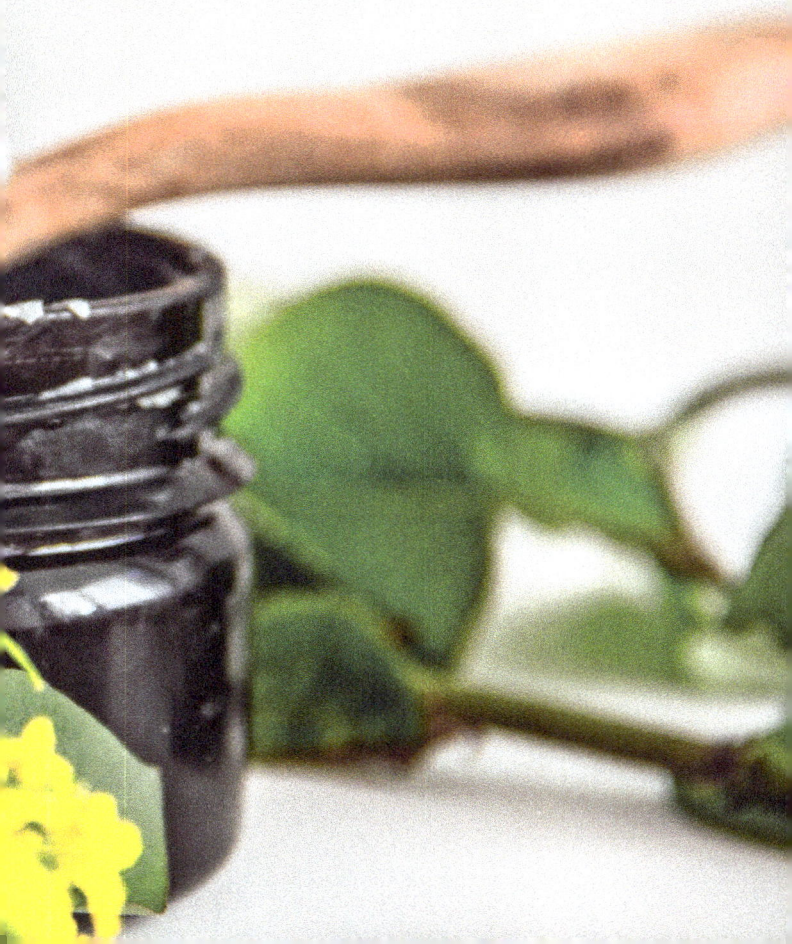

When recipes go wrong it is not always a disaster. Often they can be rescued and made right. Making mistakes is one of the best ways to learn, and sometimes the detective work in checking how things happened teaches us a lot.

Cream separates - if using Vegetal emulsifier, did you fast whisk for too long? If other emulsifiers used, did you stir or whisk for long enough until thickened? Check recipe was followed.

Grainy or gritty texture - incorrect temperature regulation before blending. Ensure water phase is at least as hot as oils phase before blending, cooler water phase will instantly solidify some of the fatty acids before they have chance to be blended to a smooth consistency. This won't harm anyone to use it, and the gritty solid fatty components will melt on skin contact, but it is unpleasant to use unless someone wants an exfoliating effect! Can be caused by insufficient stirring on cooling, or temperature fluctuations in storage. Can usually be rescued by re-melting and stirring to cool again. Add 1% extra emulsifier to ensure prevention on the remelt.

Mould - this can happen over time, and all sorts of different types of mould can grow, pink, green, black, and may be caused by inaccurate preservation methods, closing the lid whilst still warm causing condensation and damp, insufficient air tight lid, or insufficient hygiene of container. Cannot be salvaged so needs discarding.

Oily or watery pooling on the surface - inadequate blending or stopping whisking too soon.

Unpleasant smell - sometimes along with the colour of the cream darkening. This could be rancidity of the oils if it smells off and it is quite old. It can't be rectified so needs to be discarded.

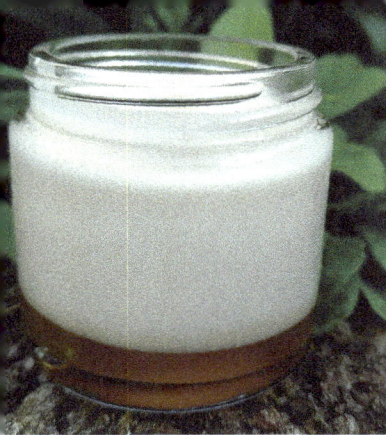

Image left. This cream shows separation of watery lower layer, and fatty upper layer. This can be due to incorrect temperature before blending, error in weighing ingredients, or incorrect whisking technique with Vegetal emulsifier.

Image right. This balm is gritty and granular. This can be caused by insufficient stirring on cooling, or temperature fluctuations in storage. This can usually be rescued by re-melting and stirring to cool again.

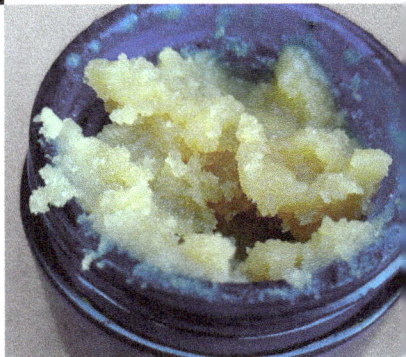

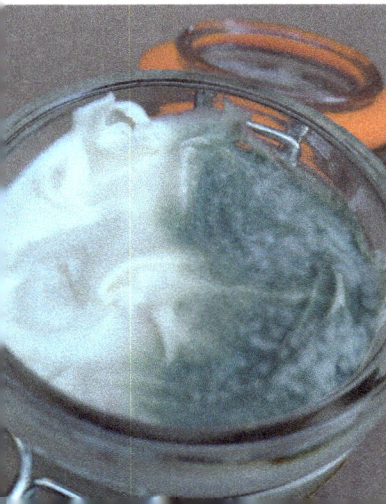

Image right. A vigorous growth of mould on this cream could be caused by inaccurate preservation methods, closing the lid whilst still warm causing condensation and damp, insufficient air tight lid, insufficient hygiene of container. This cannot be salvaged and should be discarded.

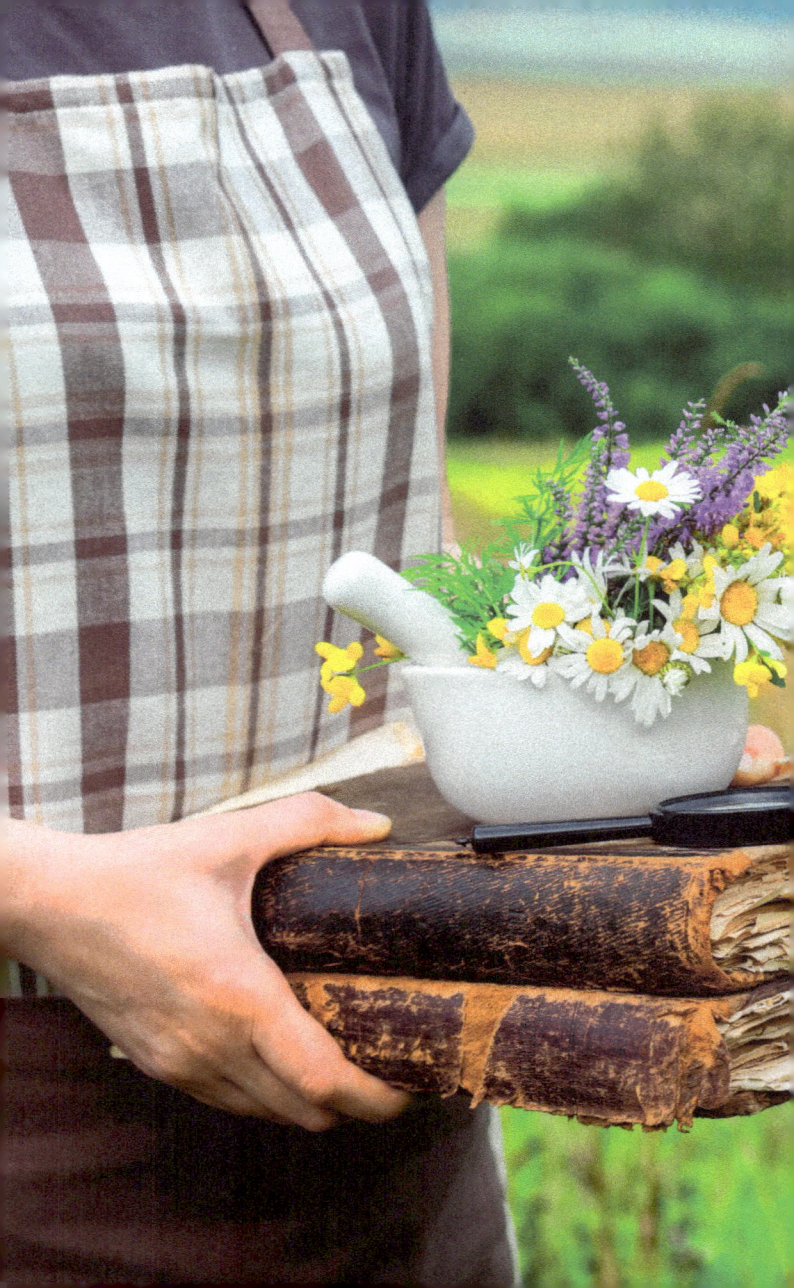

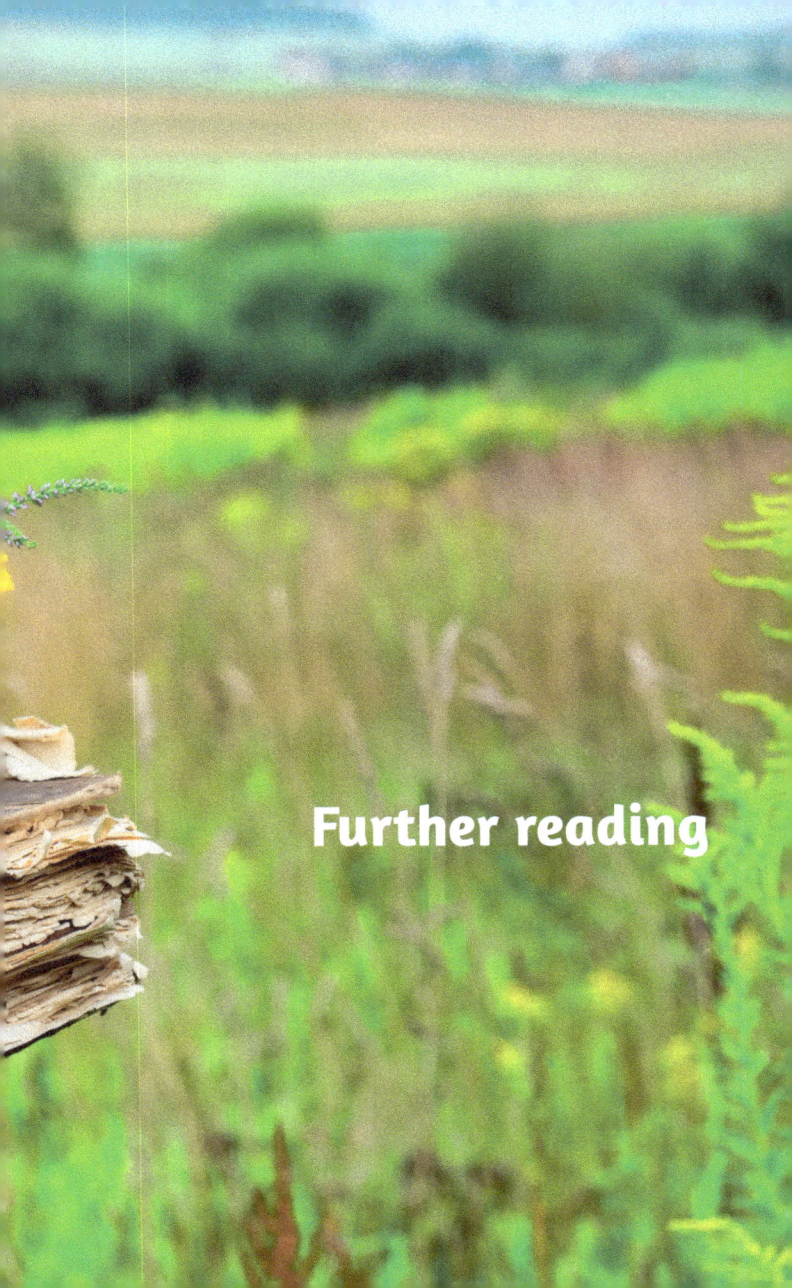

Further reading

Latin and common names of plants

Taxonomists are changing official plant names all the time, especially when genetic analysis is done and it is found plants are in different binomial families to that first categorised, such as Rosemary now being closely related to Sage, so classed as Salvia. These are accurate to the best of my knowledge at the time of writing, apologies for any that may be wrong.

Latin name	Common name
Achillea millefolium	Yarrow
Aesculus hippocastanum	Horse chestnut/ conker
Aloe vera	Aloe barbadensis
Althaea officinalis	Marshmallow
Arctostaphylos uva ursi	Bearberry
Anthemis	Roman Chamomile
Avena sativa	Oat
Bellis perennis	Daisy
Berberis aquifolium	Mahonia/Oregon Grape
Berberis vulgaris	Common Barberry
Calendula officinalis	Pot Marigold/ English Marigold
Capsicum species, various	Chilli peppers
Chamomilla recutita/ Matricaria	German Chamomile
Chelidonium majus	Greater Celandine
Commiphora myrrha	Myrrh resin
Curcuma longa	Turmeric
Echinacea angustifolia/ purpurea	Cone Flower
Filipendula ulmaria	Meadowsweet
Foeniculum vulgare	Common wild Fennel

Latin name	Common name
Fucus vesiculosis	Brown seaweed/ Bladderwrack
Gaultheria procumbens	Wintergreen
Glycyrrhiza glabra	Liquorice
Hammamelis virginiana	Witch Hazel
Hypericum perforatum	St. John's Wort
Lavendula angustifolia	Lavender
Matricaria recutita	German Chamomile
Melissa officinalis	Lemon Balm/ Bee Balm
Mentha piperita	Peppermint
Mentha spicata	Spearmint
Plantago lanceolata, major	Plantain, lance leafed/ ribwort, broad leafed
Rosa canina	Dog Rose
Salix alba	White Willow
Salvia rosmarinus	Rosemary
Silybum/Carduus marianum	Milk Thistle
Stellaria media	Chickweed
Symphytum officinalis	Comfrey, knitbone
Thymus vulgaris	Common thyme

Bibliography

• *Aromatherapy: A Practical Approach* by Vicki Pitman, Second edition, 22 Sep 2019
• *Aromadermatology: Aromatherapy in the Treatment and Care of Common Skin Conditions* by Janetta Bensouilah and Philippa Buck, 31 Oct. 2006
• *Hydrosols: The Next Aromatherapy* by Suzanne Catty, 2001

- Burlando, Bruno, Luisella Verotta, Laura Cornara, and Elisa Bottini-Massa. *Herbal Principles in Cosmetics: Properties and Mechanisms of Action*. CRC Press, 2010.
- *Aromatic Medicine* by Cathy Skipper, 2016
- Worwood, Valerie Ann. *The Fragrant Pharmacy*. New Edition. Bantam Books: Bantam, 1991.
- *The Green Witch* by Barbara Griggs, 1991

Suppliers of ingredients

Aromantic
15 Greshop Road, Greshop Industrial Estate, Forres, Moray, Scotland IV36 2GU. Tel.: 01309 696900
Website: www.aromantic.co.uk

Mystic Moments
19-20 Sandleheath Industrial Estate, Fordingbridge, Hampshire, SP6 1PA. Tel.: 01425 655555
Website: www.mysticmomentsuk.com

Naissance
Unit 11, Milland Road Industrial Estate, Milland Road, Neath, SA11 1NJ. Tel.: 01639 874637
Website: www.naissance.com
Naturally Thinking
Unit 2 Mill Lane Trading Estate, Mill Lane, Croydon, Surrey, CR0 4AA. Tel.: 020 86896489
Website: www.naturallythinking.com

The Soap Kitchen
Unit 2 Hockin Park, Caddsdown Industrial Park, Clovelly Road, EX39 3DX. Tel.: 01237 420872
Website: www.thesoapkitchen.co.uk

Baldwin & Co
171-173 Walworth Road, London, SE17 1RW.
Tel.: 020 7703 5550
Website: www.baldwins.co.uk

References

Drugs.com. 'Canesten Side Effects: Common, Severe, Long Term'. Accessed 3 December 2020. https://www.drugs.com/sfx/canesten-side-effects.html.

ScienceDaily. 'Medicine and Personal Care Products May Lead to New Pollutants in Waterways: Bacteria in Wastewater Plants Transform Widely Used Chemicals'. Accessed 3 December 2020. https://www.sciencedaily.com/releases/2019/03/190321092212.htm.

Martin, Debra, Jennifer Valdez, James Boren, and Michael Mayersohn. 'Dermal Absorption of Camphor, Menthol, and Methyl Salicylate in Humans'. *Journal of Clinical Pharmacology* 44, no. 10 (October 2004): 1151–57. https://doi.org/10.1177/0091270004268409.

Mnif, Wissem, Aziza Ibn Hadj Hassine, Aicha Bouaziz, Aghleb Bartegi, Olivier Thomas, and Benoit Roig. 'Effect of Endocrine Disruptor Pesticides: A Review'. International Journal of Environmental Research and Public Health 8, no. 6 (June 2011): 2265–2303. https://doi.org/10.3390/ijerph8062265.

Ali, S, and G Yosipovitch. 'Skin PH: From Basic SciencE to Basic Skin Care'. *Acta Dermato Venereologica* 93, no. 3 (2013): 261–67. https://doi.org/10.2340/00015555-1531.

Waller, Jeanette M., and Howard I. Maibach. 'Age and Skin Structure and Function, a Quantitative Approach (I): Blood Flow, PH, Thickness, and Ultrasound Echogenicity'. *Skin Research and Technology: Official Journal of International Society for Bioengineering and the Skin (ISBS) [and] International Society for Digital Imaging of Skin (ISDIS) [and] International Society for Skin Imaging (ISSI)* 11, no. 4 (November 2005): 221–35. https://doi.org/10.1111/j.0909-725X.2005.00151.x.

Blaak, Jürgen, Richard Wohlfart, and Nanna Schürer. 'Treatment of Aged Skin with a PH 4 Skin Care Product Normalizes Increased Skin Surface PH and Improves Barrier Function: Results of a Pilot Study'. *Journal of Cosmetics, Dermatological Sciences and Applications* 1 (1 January 2011): 50–58. https://doi.org/10.4236/jcdsa.2011.13009.

Burlando, Bruno, Luisella Verotta, Laura Cornara, and Elisa Bottini-Massa. *Herbal Principles in Cosmetics: Properties and Mechanisms of Action*. CRC Press, 2010.

Heggers, John P., John Cottingham, Jean Gusman, Lee Reagor, Lana McCoy, Edith Carino, Robert Cox, Jian-Gang Zhao, and Lana Reagor. 'The Effectiveness of Processed Grapefruit-Seed Extract as an Antibacterial Agent: II. Mechanism of Action and in Vitro Toxicity'. *Journal of Alternative and*

Complementary Medicine (New York, N.Y.) 8, no. 3 (June 2002): 333–40. https://doi.org/10.1089/10755530260128023.

Chemistry Stack Exchange. 'Solutions - Does Glycerin Promote Bacterial Growth the Same as Water?' Accessed 14 August 2020. https://chemistry.stackexchange.com/questions/46843/does-glycerin-promote-bacterial-growth-the-same-as-water.

The Dermatology Review. 'Should You Use a Vitamin E Cream?', 17 November 2013. https://thedermreview.com/vitamin-e-cream/.

Nieto, Gema, Gaspar Ros, and Julián Castillo. 'Antioxidant and Antimicrobial Properties of Rosemary (Rosmarinus Officinalis, L.): A Review'. *Medicines* 5, no. 3 (4 September 2018). https://doi.org/10.3390/medicines5030098.

European Commission' Perfume Allergies - Introduction. Accessed 14 August 2020. https://ec.europa.eu/health/scientific_committees/opinions_layman/perfume-allergies/en/index.htm.

Díaz-Maroto, M. Consuelo, M. Soledad Pérez-Coello, and M. Dolores Cabezudo. 'Supercritical Carbon Dioxide Extraction of Volatiles from Spices: Comparison with Simultaneous Distillation–Extraction'. *Journal of Chromatography* A 947, no. 1 (15 February 2002): 23–29. https://doi.org/10.1016/S0021-9673(01)01585-0.
es/en/l-3/1-introduction.htm.

'Essential Oil Safety : Aromatherapy Trade Council'. Accessed 14 August 2020. https://www.a-t-c.org.uk/safety-matters/essential-oil-safety/.

Díaz-Maroto, M. Consuelo, M. Soledad Pérez-Coello, and M. Dolores Cabezudo. 'Supercritical Carbon Dioxide Extraction of Volatiles from Spices: Comparison with Simultaneous Distillation–Extraction'. *Journal of Chromatography* A 947, no. 1 (15 February 2002): 23–29. https://doi.org/10.1016/S0021-9673(01)01585-0.

'The Forgotten Therapeutic Applications of Castor Oil | Clinical Education'. Accessed 14 August 2020. https://www.clinicaleducation.org/resources/reviews/the-forgotten-therapeutic-applications-of-castor-oil/.

Heggers, John P., John Cottingham, Jean Gusman, Lee Reagor, Lana McCoy, Edith Carino, Robert Cox, Jian-Gang Zhao, and Lana Reagor. 'The Effectiveness of Processed Grapefruit-Seed Extract as an Antibacterial Agent: II. Mechanism of Action and in Vitro Toxicity'. *Journal of Alternative and Complementary Medicine* (New York, N.Y.) 8, no. 3 (June 2002): 333–40. https://doi.org/10.1089/10755530260128023.

Guarrera, M., L. Turbino, and A. Rebora. 'The Anti-Inflammatory Activity of Azulene'. *Journal of the European Academy of Dermatology and Venereology* 15, no. 5 (2001): 486–87. https://doi.org/10.1046/j.1468-3083.2001.00340.x.

Suter, Andy, Silvia Bommer, and Jordan Rechner. 'Treatment of Patients with Venous Insufficiency with Fresh Plant Horse Chestnut Seed Extract: A Review of 5 Clinical Studies'. *Advances in Therapy* 23, no. 1 (February 2006): 179–90. https://doi.org/10.1007/BF02850359.

Bonaterra, Gabriel A., Kevin Bronischewski, Pascal Hunold, Hans Schwarzbach, Ennio-U. Heinrich, Careen Fink, Heba Aziz-Kalbhenn, Jürgen Müller, and Ralf Kinscherf. 'Anti-Inflammatory and Anti-Oxidative Effects of Phytohustil® and Root Extract of Althaea Officinalis L. on Macrophages in Vitro'. *Frontiers in Pharmacology* 11 (17 March 2020). https://doi.org/10.3389/fphar.2020.00290.

ScienceDaily. 'Natural Ingredients Used in New Topical Treatments for Hyperpigmentation: Dermatologists Explains'. Accessed 16 August 2020. https://www.sciencedaily.com/releases/2014/03/140321094703.htm.

Sobhan, Mohammadreza, Mahsa Hojati, Seyed-Yaser Vafaie, Davoud Ahmadimoghaddam, Younes Mohammadi, and Maryam Mehrpooya. 'The Efficacy of Colloidal Oatmeal Cream 1% as Add-on Therapy in the Management of Chronic Irritant Hand Eczema: A Double-Blind Study'. *Clinical, Cosmetic and Investigational Dermatology* 13 (25 March 2020): 241–51. https://doi.org/10.2147/CCID.S246021.

Brinker, Francis. 'Psoriasis Treatment with Oregon Grape Extracts' 6, no. 1 (2005): 4.

Colombo, Elisa, Enrico Sangiovanni, Michele D'Ambrosio, Enrica Bosisio, Alexandru Ciocarlan, Marco Fumagalli, Antonio Guerriero, Petru Harghel, and Mario Dell'Agli. 'A Bio-Guided Fractionation to Assess the Inhibitory Activity of Calendula Officinalis L. on the NF-KB Driven Transcription in Human Gastric Epithelial Cells'. *Evidence-Based Complementary and Alternative Medicine : ECAM* 2015 (2015). https://doi.org/10.1155/2015/727342.

Nicolaus; ResearchGate. 'In Vitro Studies to Evaluate the Wound Healing Properties of Calendula Officinalis Extracts | Request PDF'. Accessed 29 August 2020. https://doi.org/10.1016/j.jep.2016.12.006.

Saini, Pragtipal, Nouf Al-Shibani, Jun Sun, Weiping Zhang, Fengyu Song, Karen S. Gregson, and L. Jack Windsor. 'Effects of Calendula Officinalis on Human Gingival Fibroblasts'. *Homeopathy: The Journal of the Faculty of Homeopathy* 101, no. 2 (April 2012): 92–98. https://doi.org/10.1016/j.homp.2012.02.003.

'Capsaicin - an Overview | ScienceDirect Topics'. Accessed 13 October 2020. https://www.sciencedirect.com/topics/pharmacology-toxicology-and-pharmaceutical-science/capsaicin.

Jørgensen, Mette Rose, and Anne Marie Lynge Pedersen. 'Analgesic Effect of Topical Oral Capsaicin Gel in Burning Mouth Syndrome'. *Acta Odontologica Scandinavica* 75, no. 2 (March 2017): 130–36. https://doi.org/10.1080/00016357.2016.1269191.

Chrubasik, S., T. Weiser, and B. Beime. 'Effectiveness and Safety of Topical Capsaicin Cream in the Treatment of Chronic Soft Tissue Pain'. *Phytotherapy Research: PTR* 24, no. 12 (December 2010): 1877–85. https://doi.org/10.1002/ptr.3335.

Merfort, I., J. Heilmann, U. Hagedorn-Leweke, and B. C. Lippold. 'In Vivo Skin Penetration Studies of Camomile Flavones'. *Die Pharmazie* 49, no. 7 (July 1994): 509–11.

Alotaibi, Ghada. 'AN IN-VITRO STUDY TO TEST ANTIMICROBIAL EFFECTS OF COMMIPHORA MYRRHA IN COMPARISON TO BIOCIDES', n.d., 5.

Maryam Hajhashemi, Zinat Ghanbari, Minoo Movahedi, Mahmoud Rafieian, Atefeh Keivani & Fedyeh Haghollahi (2018) The effect of *Achillea millefolium* and *Hypericum perforatum* ointments on episiotomy wound healing in primiparous women, The Journal of Maternal-Fetal & Neonatal Medicine, 31:1, 63-69, DOI: 10.1080/14767058.2016.1275549

Shin, Jae Young, Denis Nchang Che, Byoung Ok Cho, Hyun Ju Kang, Jisu Kim, and Seon Il Jang. 'Commiphora Myrrha Inhibits Itch-associated Histamine and IL-31 Production in Stimulated Mast Cells'. *Experimental and Therapeutic Medicine* 18, no. 3 (1 September 2019): 1914–20. https://doi.org/10.3892/etm.2019.7721.

ResearchGate. '(PDF) Antifungal Activity of Commiphora Myrrha L. against Some Air Fungi'. Accessed 7 September 2020. https://www.researchgate.net/publication/287540286_Antifungal_activity_of_Commiphora_myrrha_L_against_some_air_fungi.

Fujimura, Tsutomu, Kazue Tsukahara, Shigeru Moriwaki, Takashi Kitahara, Tomohiko Sano, and Yoshinori Takema. 'Treatment of Human Skin with an Extract of Fucus Vesiculosus Changes Its Thickness and Mechanical Properties'. *Journal of Cosmetic Science* 53, no. 1 (February 2002): 1–9.

Michel, Piotr, Sebastian Granica, Anna Magiera, Karolina Rosińska, Małgorzata Jurek, Łukasz Poraj, and Monika Anna Olszewska. 'Salicylate and Procyanidin-Rich Stem Extracts of Gaultheria Procumbens L. Inhibit Pro-Inflammatory Enzymes and Suppress Pro-Inflammatory and Pro-Oxidant Functions of Human Neutrophils Ex Vivo'. *International Journal of Molecular Sciences* 20, no. 7 (9 April 2019). https://doi.org/10.3390/ijms20071753.

Michel, Piotr, Anna Dobrowolska, Agnieszka Kicel, Aleksandra Owczarek, Agnieszka Bazylko, Sebastian Granica, Jakub P. Piwowarski, and Monika A. Olszewska. 'Polyphenolic Profile, Antioxidant and Anti-Inflammatory Activity of Eastern Teaberry (Gaultheria Procumbens L.) Leaf Extracts'. *Molecules* 19, no. 12 (8 December 2014): 20498–520. https://doi.org/10.3390/molecules191220498.

Khar, Ashok, A. Mubarak Ali, B. V. V. Pardhasaradhi, Ch. Varalakshmi, Rana Anjum, and A. Leela Kumari. 'Induction of Stress Response Renders Human Tumor Cell Lines Resistant to Curcumin-Mediated Apoptosis: Role of Reactive Oxygen Intermediates'. *Cell Stress & Chaperones* 6, no. 4 (October 2001): 368–76.

Siracusa, Laura, Antonella Saija, Mariateresa Cristani, Francesco Cimino, Manuela D'Arrigo, Domenico Trombetta, Felice Rao, and Giuseppe Ruberto. 'Phytocomplexes from Liquorice (Glycyrrhiza Glabra L.) Leaves — Chemical Characterization and Evaluation of Their Antioxidant, Anti-Genotoxic and Anti-Inflammatory Activity'. *Fitoterapia* 82, no. 4 (1 June 2011): 546–56. https://doi.org/10.1016/j.fitote.2011.01.009.

Saeedi, M., K. Morteza-Semnani, and M.-R. Ghoreishi. 'The Treatment of Atopic Dermatitis with Licorice Gel'. *The Journal of Dermatological Treatment* 14, no. 3 (September 2003): 153–57. https://doi.org/10.1080/09546630310014369.

ResearchGate. '(PDF) Glabrene and Isoliquiritigenin as Tyrosinase Inhibitors from Licorice Roots'. Accessed 8 September 2020. https://doi.org/10.1021/jf020935u.

Mackay, Douglas. 'Hemorrhoids and Varicose Veins: A Review of Treatment Options'. *Alternative Medicine Review : A Journal of Clinical Therapeutic* 6 (1 May 2001): 126–40.

Çobanoğlu, Asuman, and Merdiye Şendir. 'The Effect of Hypericum Perforatum Oil on the Healing Process in the Care of Episiotomy Wounds: A Randomized Controlled Trial'. *European Journal of Integrative Medicine* 34 (1 February 2020): 100995. https://doi.org/10.1016/j.eujim.2019.100995.

Clewell, Amy, Matt Barnes, John Endres, Mansoor Ahmed, and Daljit Ghambeer. 'Efficacy and Tolerability Assessment of a Topical Formulation Containing Copper Sulfate and Hypericum Perforatum on Patients with Herpes Skin Lesions: A Comparative, Randomized Controlled Trial'. *Journal of Drugs in Dermatology : JDD* 11 (1 February 2012): 209–15.

Mazzanti, G., L. Battinelli, C. Pompeo, A. M. Serrilli, R. Rossi, I. Sauzullo, F. Mengoni, and V. Vullo. 'Inhibitory Activity of Melissa Officinalis L. Extract on Herpes Simplex Virus Type 2 Replication'. *Natural Product Research* 22, no. 16 (2008): 1433–40. https://doi.org/10.1080/14786410802075939.

Elsaie, Lotfy T, Abdelraouf M El Mohsen, Ibrahim M Ibrahim, Mahmoud H Mohey-Eddin, and Mohamed L Elsaie. 'Effectiveness of Topical Peppermint Oil on Symptomatic Treatment of Chronic Pruritus'. *Clinical, Cosmetic and Investigational Dermatology* 9 (11 October 2016): 333–38. https://doi.org/10.2147/CCID.S116995.

Keshavarzian, Sekine, and Nahid Shahgholian. 'Comparison of the Effect of Topical Application of Rosemary and Menthol for Musculoskeletal Pain in Hemodialysis Patients'. *Iranian Journal of Nursing and Midwifery Research* 22 (1 November 2017): 436. https://doi.org/10.4103/ijnmr.IJNMR_163_16.

Panahi, Yunes, Mohsen Taghizadeh, Eisa Tahmasbpour Marzony, and Amirhossein Sahebkar. 'Rosemary Oil vs Minoxidil 2% for the Treatment of Androgenetic Alopecia: A Randomized Comparative Trial'. *Skinmed* 13, no. 1 (February 2015): 15–21.

Muhammad Bahrain Adom, Muhammad Taher, Muhammad Fathiy Mutalabisin, Mohamad Shahreen Amri, Muhammad Badri Abdul Kudos, Mohd Wan Azizi Wan Sulaiman, Pinaki Sengupta, & Deny Susanti. 'Chemical constituents and medical benefits of plantago major' *Biomedicine & Pharmacotherapy* 96 (December 2017): 348-360. doi: 10.1016/j.biopha.2017.09.152. https://pubmed.ncbi.nlm.nih.gov/29028587/

Jowkar, Farideh, Hamid Godarzi, and Mohammad Mahdi Parvizi. 'Can We Consider Silymarin as a Treatment Option for Vitiligo? A Double-Blind Controlled Randomized Clinical Trial of Phototherapy plus Oral Silybum Marianum Product versus Phototherapy Alone'. *The Journal of Dermatological Treatment* 31, no. 3 (May 2020): 256–60. https://doi.org/10.1080/09546634.2019.1595506.

Vostálová, Jitka, Eva Tinková, David Biedermann, Pavel Kosina, Jitka Ulrichová, and Alena Rajnochová Svobodová. 'Skin Protective Activity of Silymarin and Its Flavonolignans'. *Molecules* 24, no. 6 (14 March 2019). https://doi.org/10.3390/molecules24061022.

Koll, R., M. Buhr, R. Dieter, H. Pabst, H. G. Predel, O. Petrowicz, B. Giannetti, S. Klingenburg, and C. Staiger. 'Efficacy and Tolerance of a Comfrey Root Extract (Extr. Rad. Symphyti) in the Treatment of Ankle Distorsions: Results of a Multicenter, Randomized, Placebo-Controlled, Double-Blind Study'. *Phytomedicine: International Journal of Phytotherapy and Phytopharmacology* 11, no. 6 (September 2004): 470–77. https://doi.org/10.1016/j.phymed.2004.02.001.

Cornaghi, Laura, Francesca Arnaboldi, Rossella Calò, Federica Landoni, William Franz Baruffaldi Preis, Laura Marabini, and Elena Donetti. 'Effects of UV Rays and Thymol/Thymus Vulgaris L. Extract in an Ex Vivo Human Skin Model: Morphological and Genotoxicological Assessment'. *Cells Tissues Organs* 201, no. 3 (2016): 180–92. https://doi.org/10.1159/000444361.

ResearchGate. '(PDF) Antimicrobial Activity of Topical Formulations Containing Thymus Vulgaris Essential Oil on Major Pathogens Causing Skin Diseases'. Accessed 9 September 2020. https://doi.org/10.4314/epj.v26i2.43041.

Salehzadeh, Ali, Mahsa Sadat, Hashemi Doulabi, Bita Sohrabnia, and Amir Jalali. 'The Effect of Thyme (Thymus Vulgaris) Extract on the Expression of NorA Efflux Pump Gene in Clinical Strains of Staphylococcus Aureus', *Journal of Genetic Resources*, 1 January 2018, 26–36. https://doi.org/10.22080/jgr.2018.13900.1099.

Zaman, Su, and N Akhtar. 'Effect of Turmeric (Curcuma Longa Zingiberaceae) Extract Cream on Human Skin Sebum Secretion'. *Tropical Journal of Pharmaceutical Research* 12, no. 5 (29 October 2013): 665–69. https://doi.org/10.4314/tjpr.v12i5.1

About the author

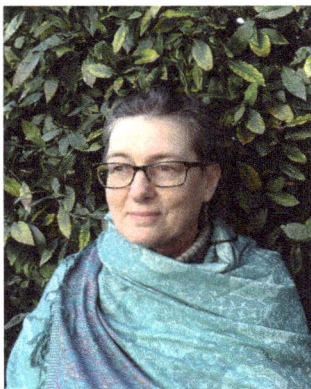

Dawn is a medical herbalist who graduated from the University of East London in 2011. She lives on the South West coast of Devon and has a particular interest in coastal herbs and medicinal wild plants including seaweed. She runs regular foraging walks in her home town of Torquay and surrounding areas. She makes many of her own herbal medicines and specialises in making medicinal creams for her practice.

Previously she worked in an organic heritage garden, and has studied and taken various courses in horticulture and herbs.

She has also worked as herbal advisor in a local independent health food shop in addition to developing the Green Wyse range of natural vegan body care products which are sold online and in many shops throughout the UK.

Alongside her herbal practice Dawn writes herb related articles for various magazines, and offers herbal student mentoring and clinic training days.

WITH A LOVE FOR BOOKS

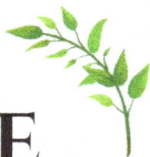

With a large range of imprints, from herbalism, selfsufficiency, physical and mental wellbeing, food, memoirs and many more, Herbary Books is shaped by the passion for writing and bringing innovative ideas close to our readers.

All our authors put their hearts into their books and as publishers we just lend a helping hand to bring their creation to life.

Thank you to our authors and to you, dear reader.

Discover and purchase all our books on

WWW.HERBARYBOOKS.COM

HERBARYBOOKS